Jo.

3.95?

Kin Holmes.

Guidelines on Patient Care in Radiography

107.
100

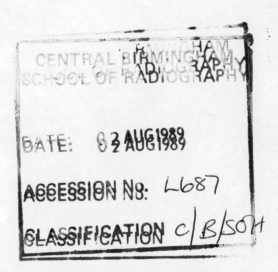

Guidelines on Patient Care in Radiography

Christine Gunn TDCR
Deputy Principal,
Derbyshire Royal Infirmary School of Radiography

Christine S Tozer TDCR
Deputy Principal,
Hogarth School of Radiotherapy,
Nottingham

Foreword by

Shirley Williams TDCR
Radiotherapy Principal,
School of Radiotherapy,
Newcastle Upon Tyne

CHURCHILL LIVINGSTONE
EDINBURGH LONDON MELBOURNE AND NEW YORK 1982

CHURCHILL LIVINGSTONE
Medical Division of Longman Group Limited

Distributed in the United States of America by
Churchill Livingstone Inc., 1560 Broadway,
New York, N.Y. 10036, and by associated companies,
branches and representatives throughout the world.

First published 1982
  Reprinted 1984

ISBN 0 443 02545 2

British Library Cataloguing in Publication Data
Gunn, Christine
    Guidelines on patient care in radiography.
    1. Diagnosis, Radioscopic
    I. Title II. Tozer, Christine S.
    616.07'57'024613   RC78

Library of Congress Catalog Card Number
Gunn, Christine.
    Guidelines in patient care in radiography.
    Includes index.
    1. Radiography, Medical. 2. Radiotherapy.
3. Radiologic technologists. 4. Nursing.
I. Tozer, Christine S. II. Title. [DNLM:
1. Hospital departments—Organization and
administration—Handbooks. 2. Patients—Handbooks.
3. Radiography—Handbooks. 4. Radiotherapy—
Handbooks.   WN 200 G977 g]
RC78.G86   616.07'57   81-21700
                                         AACR2

Printed in Singapore by Huntsmen Offset Printing Pte Ltd

Foreword

The writers of this book have a great deal of experience both in the clinical and teaching side of their profession and this is shown quite clearly by the high standard of information contained in it.

I highly recommend this concise little book for use by therapeutic and diagnostic student radiographers and radiographers both as a guide to the care of the patient in the X-ray and Radiotherapy Department and also as a help towards passing the Care of the Patient and Hospital Practice section of the D.C.R. examination.

The new syllabus set by the College of Radiographers now has a section on psychological aspects regarding the care of the patient and I am glad to see this important aspect of the radiographer's work so adequately covered in this book. Not only to the radiographers do I recommend it but also to all the staff working with or having contact with patients in an X-ray or Radiotherapy Department.

Newcastle upon Tyne 1982   S. Williams

Preface

This book was written as a precise reference guide to the care of the patient in the X-ray and Radiotherapy Departments.

Our aim is to provide essential information which may be of use, not only to student radiographers and radiographers but also to X-ray and Radiotherapy nurses and other paramedical staff having contact with patients.

We anticipate that student radiographers will use the guide alongside more detailed texts which, together with the relevant practical experience, will help to provide the student radiographer with a sound basis on which to develop a high standard of patient care.

The 25 chapters contain information on all aspects of patient care. At the beginning of each chapter, an introduction outlines the reasons why the information which follows has been included. It is difficult to know how much information is necessary (or unnecessary) and we have tried to produce a book which achieves a balance between a purely factual notebook and a detailed textbook.

1982   C.G.
                                                                     C.S.T.

Acknowledgements

We would like to thank the following people who have read and constructively criticised the manuscript, Mr H.B. Bentley, Principal, School of Radiography, The General Infirmary, Leeds; Mrs S. Williams, Principal, School of Radiotherapy, Newcastle; Mrs P.L. Humphreys, Staff Nurse, Mansfield General Hospital; Mrs L. Smith, Senior Radiographer, Derbyshire Royal Infirmary and Mrs M. Smith, Clinical Instructor, Hogarth School of Radiotherapy, Nottingham.

Grateful thanks are also given to Miss V. Seagrave, Deputy Principal, Nottinghamshire Area School of Radiography for her contribution in the Ultrasound and Nuclear Medicine section; Mr H. Beckett, District Fire Prevention Officer, Derbyshire Royal Infirmary for the section on Fire prevention; Dr A.L.M. Piotrowicz, Consultant Radiologist, Derbyshire Royal Infirmary for his comments on the section involving contrast agents and patient preparation for diagnostic procedures and Mr D. Graham, Principal, Grampian School of Radiography, Aberdeen for assistance with the sections on Nuclear Medicine and Nuclear Magnetic Resonance.

We would also like to thank the College of Radiographers for giving us permission to use abstracts from the Examiners' comments from the Care of the Patient and Hospital Practice papers.

All the artwork for this book has been drawn by Dr D.A. Gunn to whom the authors are extremely grateful as the illustrations would not have been possible without his help.

C.G.
C.S.T.

Acknowledgments

Contents

1

Departmental organisation and procedure

INTRODUCTION

The aim of this section is to provide the student radiographer with information regarding general departmental procedures. It is important that the student is aware that the practical running of hospital departments requires an efficient hospital team of which they have become a member. Emphasis must be placed on gaining practical experience within their own departments and the guidelines set out in this chapter should help the student to have an understanding of departmental organisation and the importance of record keeping.

At the end of this section are notes concerning medico-legal aspects of hospital administration.

Whilst we feel that to burden students with complicated legal procedures and laws is unnecessary, nevertheless a basic appreciation of medico-legal aspects regarding hospital personnel and patients in the department should be within the capabilities of student radiographers.

WAITING AREAS

When planning waiting areas the following points should be considered:

Sufficient area to accommodate patients and 'friends'
Separate areas for children/badly injured/ward patients
Sufficient comfortable chairs and small tables
Well ventilated, no draughts, suitable temperature
Pleasant decor
Clean magazines, goldfish, piped music may be available
Toys for children (washable – to reduce the likelihood of infection)
Toilet facilities – adjacent and well signposted

Refreshments available or instructions where they can be obtained.
Receptionist available to assist the patients

APPOINTMENT SYSTEMS

Required to:
Minimise patient waiting time
Ensure full use of staff and equipment
When booking an appointment –
For In Patients avoid
Meal times
Doctors ward rounds
Drug administration rounds
Visiting time
For Out Patients consider
The distance the patient has to travel and the time it may take
Use of hostel accommodation for radiotherapy patients
If the patient is on 'shift work'
If the patient has dependants (young children, etc.)
If the the appointment can be arranged to coincide with other hospital visits
If an ambulance will be required
If an ambulance escort will be required
Any clinical features e.g. a strict schedule is required for diabetic patients

DIAGNOSTIC X-RAY EXAMINATION REQUEST FORMS

Ideally these should give the following information

Patient details
Full name
Address
Hospital registration number
Age/date of birth
X-ray number
Occupation
Sex
Married/single/widowed
Method of transport from the ward e.g. if a trolley is required
Ward/Out patient

Date of last menstrual period
Date and place of previous radiographs

Departmental information
Radiographic examination requested
Doctor's signature
Consultant in charge of the case
Any clinical features/diagnosis
Observe/ignore 10 day rule
Number of films for reporting
Radiographer's signature
Exposure factors used
Space for the Radiologist's report

The above information is required to ensure that the correct patient is radiographed and any previous radiographs/reports can be obtained. The person referring the patient and the radiographer responsible for the radiographs can be contacted if necessary.

RADIOTHERAPY HISTORY

Patients are assigned a radiotherapy case number and the history may be colour coded to show the year that treatment commenced. Confidential reports are required of:

Patient diagnosis and associated literature
Patient background history
Pathology reports
X-ray reports etc.
Correspondence concerning patients
Ward details for In patients or Radiotherapy hostel patients
Drug prescriptions
Patients consent to treatment form

RADIOTHERAPY PRESCRIPTIONS

Ideally they should give the following information

Patient details
Full name
Hospital number
Diagnosis
In/Out patient

Treatment details
Treatment machine
Beam energy
Focus to skin distance
Field size
Position of fields
Beam direction devices
Wedges
Compensators
Treatment plan
Percentage depth dose at the tumour
Skin dose
Applied dose
Interfield distance
Special instructions e.g. blood counts to be undertaken
Information recorded daily by the radiographer during treatment
Summary of treatment on completion

DEPARTMENTAL STATISTICS

Diagnostic
Records are kept concerning
   Patient attendances – In/Out patients
   The number of radiographic examinations undertaken
   The number of X-ray units
Unit values are based on the time required to undertake specific examinations and they are used to assess
   Staffing levels
   Film requirements
   Chemicals required
   Drugs required
   Equipment required
   Future planning of the department
As the following patients and examinations take longer to perform, additional units are given for
   Blind patients
   Children (under the age of 6)
   Deaf patients
   Patients with language difficulties
   Intoxicated patients
   Mentally ill patients
   Mentally handicapped patients
   Physically crippled patients

Unconscious patients (other than anaesthetised)
Mobile/portable examinations
Operating theatre work
Visits to other hospitals
Domiciliary visits

All records are kept during the patient's lifetime, in some hospitals after 5 years the notes are microfilmed for ease of storage.

Radiographs are kept for 7 years (soon to be changed to 21 years) and are then sent for silver recovery.

Radiotherapy

Records are kept concerning
Number of new cases per year
Total number of treated cases per year
Number of radiation fields applied per year
Number of chemotherapy cases per year
Number of biopsies performed per year.

The above records are kept so as to predict:
A percentage workload increase/decrease
Correct staff establishment
Correct treatment machine establishment

The records may also be used for research purposes.

Storage of radiographs

Each radiograph should give the following information, (preferably photographed on)
Patient's name
Hospital
The date the radiographic examination was undertaken
An anatomical marker
Patient identification number

Radiographs are stored in paper envelopes which carry details of
Patient's name
X-ray number
The radiographic examinations which have been performed

Radiographs can be filed under
X-ray registration number
The date of birth of the patient
The patient's name (in alphabetical order)

Radiographs should be stored
Away from direct heat
Away from damp
In an area of constant temperature

MEDICO-LEGAL ASPECTS

Accidents in the department

Hospital personnel should always be on their guard as most accidents are preventable. Patient injury could be caused by –

Radiation equipment
  Mechanical hazards
  Irradiation hazards
  Electrical hazards

Accessory equipment
  Treatment/X-ray couch
  Wheelchairs
  Cones/cassettes/grids
  Foot stools

Departmental
  Slippery material on the floor
  Dangerous materials e.g. broken glass
  Poor lighting
  Incorrect storage of articles

Patient care procedures
  Incorrect identification of patients
  Incorrect treatment/investigations of patients
  Incorrect drug administration to patients
  Incorrect handling of patients
  Inadequate hygiene standards – cross infection

Accidents involving equipment and departmental design apply equally well to hospital personnel.

Accident routine
Attend to the patient
Report to the head of department
Inform medical officer if necessary
Fill in an accident form (see chapter on First Aid)

HEALTH AND SAFETY AT WORK ACT

Instituted in 1974.
Applies to all persons at work (except domestic employees in private households).

Principal objectives
  To involve all staff at the work place and to create an awareness of the importance of achieving a high standard of health and safety

It is the duty of everyone to take reasonable care for health and safety

Student radiographers should

Be aware of the work of their safety representative

Know the safety policy of their own employing authority

Be aware of all possible hazards within a department

Be able to correctly fill in the accident forms

Staff working in X-ray or Radiotherapy Departments should integrate the Health and Safety Policy with the Code of Practice for the protection of Persons against Ionizing Radiations arising from Medical and Dental Use.

N.B. Should an accident occur due to negligence on the part of an individual they may not be covered by the employing authority.

PROFESSIONAL ATTITUDES

Students begining their training should be aware of the attitude towards –

Patients:

With reference to

Patient confidentiality

Care of patients before

during

after treatment/examination

Patience and understanding

Appreciation of patient problems

Other staff

Respect for other staff

Cooperation

Importance of teamwork

Punctuality

Liaison with staff in other departments

2

Hygiene

INTRODUCTION

It is essential that student radiographers understand and practice the rules relating to hygiene with regard to themselves, their patients and the working environment.

A high standard of hygiene is expected from every member of staff in the hospital and the following section is intended to help the student to develop a common sense approach to hygiene standards.

To ensure that cross-infection is kept to a minimum the following points should be considered –

Personal
Uniform coats should
   Be clean and changed when necessary
   Cover clothing
   Only be worn inside the hospital
   Be of the correct length and not too tight
Protective gowns should be worn in theatre and when handling an infectious patient
Footwear
   Shoes should be comfortable and in good repair
   Quiet, safe, protective and only worn inside the hospital
   Socks/tights should be clean
   Special shoes should be worn in the operating theatre.
Hair should be
   Either short or tied back
   Clean and tidy
   Covered completely in the operating theatre
Diet
   Should be well balanced
   Regular meals should be taken
   Regular bowel habits are to be encouraged
   Care should be taken with regard to dental hygiene

Bathing
   Reduces infection
   Refreshing and relaxing
In general
   Finger nails, short, clean, with no nail varnish
   If watches and jewellery are worn, care should be taken to ensure that there are no sharp edges which could scratch a patient
   Face masks should be worn when necessary
   Cuts on hands should be covered
   Hands washed after handling patients/dressings/bedpans/urinals/catheters/soiled instruments etc.

Patient
Clean gowns/bed linen/cubicles/X-ray room/treatment room
Disposable materials and equipment used e.g. syringes/needles/drinking receptacles/denture holders/bedpans
Hand washing facilities must be available

Equipment
Kept socially clean
Special care with equipment for use in the operating theatre
Use of washable items e.g. foam pads/covers for sandbags and bolus bags
Sterile equipment used for aseptic procedures
Use of covered receptacles for used dressings

Department
Kept socially clean
Good ventilation/air conditioning
Equipment kept in cupboards and so free from dust
Adequate washing facilities should be available
'Clean' and 'dirty' examinations kept separate
Special areas reserved for surgical trolley setting
Toilet facilities checked and cleaned regularly

3

Management of patients and patient psychology

INTRODUCTION

Throughout the training period and following on to the post qualification period, radiographers will experience a variety of patient personalities and patients with special difficulties needing extra attention.

Students will quickly be confronted by a variety of problems which will need patience and a lot of common sense. The way in which people respond towards patients depends a great deal on their own personality but with the practical guidelines of this chapter, combined with the experiences learnt in the department the student should develop both a psychological and practical competence for handling patients.

GENERAL PATIENT PSYCHOLOGY

Treat all patients with courtesy and respect
Refer to patients by name
Be polite, efficient and sympathetic
Be aware of emotional problems connected with
    Illness
    Treatment/examination procedures
    Hospitals
Be careful when coping with
    Relatives
    Racial problems in an interracial society
Be aware of physical problems associated with
    Illness
    Age
    Low level of intelligence

COMMUNICATING WITH THE PATIENT

Do we always do our best to communicate with and understand our patient's needs?

Do we
    Always give the patient enough time
    Face the patient squarely when talking or listening
    Keep good eye contact, showing interest and concern
    Create the opportunity for personal communication by adopting a
    natural stance (not with arms folded)
    Try to be at the same eye level as the patient, standing above a
    seated patient will make him feel awkward
    Bring comfort to a distressed patient by touching him – physical
    contact brings a person closer to another
    Encourage new students, not accustomed to physical patient
    contact, to help with the lifting of patients
    Share a sense of humour with our patients
    Encourage patients to talk of their fears and problems by asking
    'open ended' questions e.g. 'How are you managing at home
    when the treatment is making you tired?'

If the answer to these questions is yes, then you care for your
patient.

The psychological impact of illness/cancer
The state of being in good health is something we all take for
granted. Not until this state changes, do we appreciate that our
lifestyle depends upon our continuing good health.

What problems do we have to face when our health takes a
change for the worse?

What anxieties are our patients suffering when they take their
first step into the X-ray or Radiotherapy Department?

Put yourself in their place.

General illness
What is wrong with me?
Do you know my diagnosis?
Am I going to get better?
Will I suffer any pain – with the illness
                        with the investigations?
Will I look any different?
Will I feel any different?
Why has it happened to me?
Will you answer all my questions?
Will you think of me as an individual in my own right?
Will I remember all of your instructions?
Will you think that I am stupid if I forget what you have told me?
Will I have to come again?

Cancer patients

Why has it happened to me?
Where have I got it from?
Have I really got cancer?
When am I going to die?
Will I feel any pain?
Why does the operation scar look so ugly?
Do I look ugly to you?
Why do some people avoid my questions?
Why have I heard so many conflicting stories about Radiotherapy?
Will it burn my skin?
Will it burn me inside?
Will I feel sick?
Will my hair fall out?
Will the radiation make me sterile?
Will I become radioactive?
Will I remember all my instructions?
When will I feel better?
Why was Mrs. X so ill after her treatment?
Will I have to come back for some more treatment?
Why do I have to have all these tests and investigations?
Is it true that cancer is curable?
Could I be one of the lucky ones?
Shall I start planning for the future?

General problems

Can I cope with all this?
Who will look after my children, wife, husband, parents, animals?
Should I make a will?
Who will pay the bills?
Who will do the shopping?
Who will service the car?
Will I be able to drive?
Who will explain about the tablets which I am taking?
What will I tell my family and friends?
When can I start work again?
Will I have a job to return to?
Why have people started to treat me differently?
Am I of any use?
Will my life ever be the same?
Do you now see what 'Care of the patient' is all about?

Deaf patients

Take special care when checking their identity

Make a note of their disability on the request form/treatment sheet
Use clear, slow speech
Face the patient as they may be able to lip read
Use sign language/written instructions
Always fetch a patient from the waiting area
Check the understanding of instructions by asking the patient to repeat them
Avoid unnecessary chatter which may confuse the patient
Avoid hazards e.g. approaching trolleys
Ensure the patient understands when they can leave
Check transport details
Never shout at the patient
Return deaf aids promptly (if they have been removed during the treatment/examination)

Blind patients
Respect their independence
Note the disability on request form/treatment sheet
Carefully guide the patient, avoiding obstacles
Inform the patient about the length of corridors/of any steps/if the route is either flat or sloping.
Explain procedures carefully including any noises e.g. tomographic equipment/treatment machine noise
Indicate the length of time they will be required to wait
Care with the guide dog
If the patient has to wait e.g. for an ambulance, arrange for a member of staff to speak to the patient at regular intervals to ensure he is all right.

Patient with language difficulties
Extra precautions when checking their identity
Clear, simple language if some English is understood
Possible use of an interpreter e.g. a member of staff or a relative to explain instructions
Use sign language/demonstrate
Give written instructions for future examinations/treatments

A frightened child
Avoid undue waiting
Friendly approach with extra patience
Allow plenty of time
Try to win the child's confidence
Have coloured pictures and toys available
Use discretion regarding the presence of parents

Good liaison with parents – explanation of possible side effects
Consider demonstrating on the parents (do not irradiate)
Always inform the child if any procedure is going to hurt them
Careful use of restraining/immobilisation devices
Encourage the child to look forward to future examinations/treatments
Last resort – sedation

Hemiplegic (patient is paralysed down one side)
Exercise care when lifting the patient
Special care with the paralysed side
Remove objects from the table top/treatment couch to prevent injury
Ensure limbs are on the trolley/table and are not under the patient

An unconscious patient
If possible radiograph/treat when the department is not busy
Have suction and oxygen equipment available
The emergency tray should be available
Observe the patient to ensure that:
    A clear airway is maintained
    There is no change in the skin colour
    The pulse and respiration rates are taken and recorded
Any change in condition should be reported
Speed and adaptation of technique is required
Do not leave unattended
Return to the Ward/Casualty with an escort

Care of patient valuables
Discourage patient's from bringing valuables and excess amounts of money into the hospital
Provision of a safe storage place – under lock and key
Patient and radiographer should check the contents
Patient should be issued with a receipt
Return valuables to the patient promptly
Ensure the patient signs for their return

4

Care of the unconscious and anaesthetised patient

INTRODUCTION

During the course of their work student radiographers will come into contact with unconscious and anaesthetised patients. In the diagnostic department patients may be seen directly after a major accident, or may require a general anaesthetic for more specialised examinations.

In the radiotherapy departments young children requiring a general anaesthetic and post operative patients with carcinoma of the cervix and uterus, who have had radioactive caesium inserted, may be seen.

Student radiographers should be aware of how to care for these patients and be familiar with any complications which may occur.

POSSIBLE CAUSES OF UNCONSCIOUSNESS

General anaesthetic
Brain tumour
Cardiac arrest
Cerebro vascular accident
Concussion
Diabetic coma
Drowning
Drug overdose
Epileptic fit
Fainting
Haemorrhage
Insulin coma
Poisoning

CARE OF THE UNCONSCIOUS PATIENT

Airway
Check for obstruction which may be due to vomit, false teeth etc.

If the patient is supine, lower jaw is held forward
An artificial airway may be inserted
Expired air resuscitation may be administered if required

Pulse
Check heart beat
Administer cardiac massage if required

Patient position
Place in the recovery position – unless contraindicated
Ensure the patient is kept warm
Ensure plenty of fresh air

Haemorrhage
Check for bleeding – treat as necessary
Check skin colour/respiratory rate/any change in the level of consciousness

General
Reassure the patient – hearing is the first sense to return
Give nothing by mouth
Do not leave the patient unattended
Check equipment is functioning correctly e.g. infusion sets/oxygen etc.

UNCONSCIOUS PATIENTS IN THE X-RAY DEPARTMENT

Casualty patients
Speed is essential when dealing with the patient
Do not keep the patient waiting
Have cassettes and X-ray equipment ready
Plan the order in which the radiographs are taken – to prevent undue movement of the patient e.g. all lateral projections exposed in succession
Double check the patient's identity
Do not leave the patient unattended

OPERATING THEATRE PROCEDURE

Ensure mobile X-ray unit/cassettes cleaned e.g. with suitable disinfectant
Correct clothing, mask, cap, gown, theatre shoes worn by radiographer

Check that it is the correct patient
Care taken not to contaminate sterile areas
Cover the X-ray tube head before placing over sterile field
Ask anaesthetist to control patient's respiration during exposure
Take and return films quickly

After the operation
Dispose of theatre clothing
Clean mobile X-ray unit
Check identity of films

UNCONSCIOUS PATIENTS IN THE RADIOTHERAPY DEPARTMENT

Young children are usually the only patients to be anaesthetised under the radiographers' care.

These are young children who are totally uncooperative during treatment.

A fast acting barbiturate is needed to induce narcosis.

Throughout the treatment period there should be liaison with
The radiotherapist
Department of anaesthetics
Ward staff (if child is an In patient)
Ambulance department
The parents

Ensure that:
Instructions are given about meal arrangements
Appointment time given to suit all involved in the procedure, if possible the same time each day, the first appointment in the morning is often the most suitable
Oxygen, suction and emergency drugs are available
Treatment given as quickly as possible
Provision for monitoring the heart rate during treatment is made
Quiet room for recovery period is available.

Other patients under anaesthesia
e.g. Post caesium insertion
Special unit – Cathetron

PATIENTS FOR GENERAL ANAESTHETIC

Check
Identity bracelet (on either the arm or leg)
Correct notes have arrived with the patient
Dentures removed, mouth clean
Consent form signed
Correct clothing worn

Sedated patients
Must not be left alone
Trolley should have cot sides up
Patient may require careful restraining

During the Induction of an anaesthetic
Anaesthetist should not be left alone
Staff should remain quiet
Where necessary
Assist with the intravenous injection
Check pulse and blood pressure
Pass drugs and instruments to the anaesthetist

After anaesthesia
Patient placed in recovery room if available
Oxygen, suction, emergency drugs should be available.

CARE OF THE ANAESTHETISED PATIENT

Airway
Artificial airway may be in the patient's mouth
If the patient is lying supine, hold the lower jaw forward
Check for any obstruction of the airway e.g. due to vomit, blood
or mucus

Patient position
Recovery position unless contraindicated
Check limbs are on the trolley and not trapped underneath the
patient
Ensure patient is warm and away from bright lights and noise

Skin
If the skin becomes cyanosed
Check the patient's airway

Oxygen may be required
Send for medical aid

Observations
Check and record blood pressure, pulse, temperature and respiration every 15 minutes
Report any changes
Check skin colour, report any changes

Intravenous infusions and drainage tubes
Check that infusions are working and that the tubing is not kinked or trapped

Operation/injection site
Check every 15 minutes for
   Haemorrhage
   Haematoma
   Oedema

Complications which may occur
Airway obstruction
Vomiting
Restlessness
Haemorrhage
Shock
Cardiac arrest
Respiratory failure

5

Transportation of patients

INTRODUCTION

It is necessary when moving/lifting patients to adopt a technique which is safe for the patient and can be carried out without strain to the staff. For staff, the most important aspect is the problem of placing undue strain on the spinal column.

TROLLEY PATIENTS

N.B. Patient's with fractured spines must not be moved from the trolley, except when supervised by a medical officer.

Whilst waiting
Ensure the cot sides are up
Position the trolley so that it does not cause an obstruction
Trolley should be moved by 2 members of staff

Before lifting the patient from the trolley to X-ray table or treatment couch
Give explanation and reassurance to the patient
Ensure trolley and couch locks are on
Release cot sides
Obtain enough assistance, 3 people to lift
Check there are no obstacles in the way
Ensure the X-ray tube head is not above the table/couch
Note the position of any urinary drainage bags, intravenous infusions, fractures, wounds.
Explain the procedure to the patient
Stand in a line by the trolley
If possible, fold the patient's arms over their chest
Lifters place their arms under the patient
Ensure patients's head, buttocks and legs are supported
Bend knees, back straight – lift

Patient is supported close to the lifter's body
Together walk to the table
Gently lower the patient into the correct position on the couch
Check that the patient's limbs are not trapped.

Advantages of a trolley
Stable and rigid
Area for patient's clothing
Area for oxygen cylinder and column to support infusion bags or bottles
Cot sides are available
Can be locked into position
Adjustable back rest sometimes available
Patient can be radiographed on trolleys with radiolucent tops

STRETCHER AND POLES

Canvas stretcher with 2 wooden/metal poles which slip into the canvas
Patient placed on the canvas, on a trolley, and wheeled to the department
Poles inserted in the sides of the canvas
Spreader placed between the poles to give the canvas rigidity
2 or 4 people required to lift
Explain procedure to the patient
Lift patient gently on to the table
Care that infusions, drains, catheters are not dislodged.

Advantages of the canvas
Cheap
Easy to use
Patient can be radiographed/treated on the canvas
Easier to lift heavy patients

Special considerations when radiographing patient's with radioactive caesium in situ
Make a different appointment time from other patients
Do not keep the patient waiting
Minimum time spent by the staff next to the patient's trolley
Allow nurse to attend to the care of the patient
Have the X-ray equipment ready
Return the patient to the ward as soon as possible

WHEELCHAIR PATIENTS

Place the chair at the side of the treatment couch/table
Apply brakes
Explain the procedure to the patient
Remove the footrest
Lock couch at the correct height for the patient or ensure steps are available
Two members of staff assist the patient out of the chair –
   1 holding the chair
   1 supporting the patient
Care with urinary drainage bags and catheters, fractures, wounds
Sit patient on the couch
Allow time for patient to rest
Assist patient into position on the couch
Reverse the procedure when assisting the patient off the couch.

Lifting a patient from a wheelchair to the table
Place wheelchair near the table
2 people required to assist the patient
Explain procedure to the patient
Move the patient forward –until sitting on the edge of the chair
Stand either side of the patient facing the back of the chair
Place shoulder nearest patient under the patient's axilla
Place arm nearest patient under patient's thighs
Clasp the wrist of the other lifter
Patient's arms hang over lifter's back
Support patient's back with free hand
Lifters bend knees and keeping their backs straight, lift the patient
Sit patient on table
Lift patient's legs onto the table

BED PATIENTS

To raise to a sitting position
Explain procedure to the patient
2 people are required
Stand either side of the bed, facing the head of the bed
Place forearm of arm nearest the patient under patient's axilla
Bend knees, back straight
Carefully raise patient

To move the patient up the bed
Explain the procedure to the patient
Raise the patient to the sitting position
Ask patient to bend his/her knees
Place forearm nearest the patient under the patient's axilla
Bend knees, back straight, lift the patient up the bed
At the same time patient pushes on the bed to assist (patient only asked to assist if able)

To lift the patient e.g. to place a cassette underneath
Explain procedure to the patient
3 people required, 2 to lift, 1 to position the cassette
Lifters stand at one side of the bed, the third person at the other side
Lifters bend knees, place arms under patient's shoulders and buttocks
Lift, keeping back straight
Third person positions the cassette
Patient is gently lowered
To remove the cassette – reverse the procedure

6

Inflammation and infection

INTRODUCTION

This section on inflammation and infection should be linked with the notes on hygiene, sterilisation and asepsis. In order to understand how infection can be controlled and the spread prevented it is necessary to have some basic knowledge of types of bacteria and the inflammatory process. There is no attempt to cover this vast subject in any detail because it is intended as an aid to help the student radiographer grasp the concept of what infection and sterilisation means in the confines of the clinical department.

INFLAMMATION

This is the reaction of vascular and supporting elements of tissues to various traumatic occurrences.

The inflammatory process should
  Limit the agent damaging the tissues
  Render the organisms harmless
  Repair the area of damage

Causes

Invasion by microorganisms
Mechanical trauma
Thermal trauma
Chemical trauma
Electrical trauma
Radiation trauma

Local effects of inflammation

Pain and tenderness – due to tissue sensitivity ('stretching') and pressure on sensory nerve endings
Redness and heat – dilation of blood vessels

Swelling – increased blood supply and blood flow with alteration of blood vessel walls which changes osmo regulation, allowing fluid to flow into the tissue spaces

Loss of function

Formation of pus – formed by tissue and serum fluid, cellular constituents, living and dead bacteria.

Systemic effects (if the local reaction is not contained)

Pyrexia

Anorexia

Leucocytosis

Increased pulse and respiration rate

Decreased urinary output.

Cellular reaction to infection

Increase in polymorphonuclear leucocytes – particularly neutrophils which ingest bacteria by phagocytosis

Monocytes ingest polymorphs and debris

Lymphocytes produce antibodies against invading pathogens.

Pathogens produce a complex protein around themselves – an antigen. This triggers lymphocytes to manufacture specific antibodies against the antigen.

Antitoxin can be manufactured to neutralise toxins which may be produced by some pathogens e.g. Tetanus produces a neurotoxin affecting the central nervous system.

BACTERIA

Unicellular micro-organisms, most are harmless in their natural environment.

PATHOGENS

Bacteria causing disease

Examples:

Cocci – round in shape

Arranged in clusters – Staphylococcus aureus (Fig. 6.1)

Arranged in chains – Streptococcus (Fig. 6.2)

Arranged in pairs – Diplococcus pneumonius (Fig. 6.3)

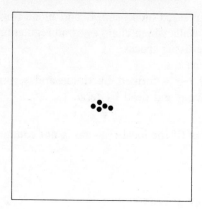

Fig. 6.1 Staphylococcus

Fig. 6.2 Streptococcus

Fig. 6.3 Diplococcus

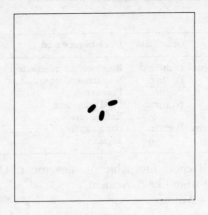

Fig. 6.4 Bacilli

Bacilli – rod shaped (Fig. 6.4)
Salmonella species
Clostridium perfrigens

Spirochaete – thready spirals (Fig. 6.5)
Treponema pallidum
Most bacteria can be gram stained
 Positive – blue stain
 Negative – red stain

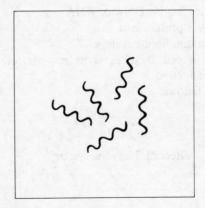

Fig. 6.5 Spirochaete

Characteristics of pathogens

Average size – 0·2 – 1·0 micron diameter 0·5–4·0 micron length
(spirochaete much longer)

Table 6.1   Gram stains

Organisms	Gram stain	Diseases produced
Staphylococcus aureus	Positive	Boils, wound infections
Streptococcus	Positive	Sore throats, tonsilitis
Diplococcus	Positive	Pneumonia
Salmonella	Negative	Food poisoning, Enteric fevers
Clostridium perfrigens	Positive	Gas gangrene
Treponema pallidum	–	Syphilis

Motility – All cocci incapable of movement. Others possess flagella allowing whip like movement.

Reproduction – Mitosis

Food requirements – Most bacteria need organic material

Oxygen requirements – Most need oxygen – aerobic bacteria without oxygen – anaerobic bacteria

Temperature requirements – Optimum temperature for most pathogens is 37°C

Spore formation – Some bacteria are capable of producing a protective outer coating which protects the bacteria from heat and disinfectants e.g. tubercle bacillus and anthrax.

VIRUSES

Consist of
  A core of nucleic acid – DNA or RNA
  Surrounded by a protein coat
  Often enclosed in a lipid envelope
When invading a cell it takes complete control, using it for growth and reproduction.
Cell destruction follows.

Types of virus
Poliomyelitis   )
) affecting Nervous system
Rabies   )

Smallpox   )
)
Chickenpox   ) affecting Skin
)
Measles   )

Viral carcinogenesis
Some viruses are thought to have tumour inducing properties. Ep-

stein-Barr virus (DNA virus) plus malaria is thought to produce Birkitt's lymphoma which is endemic in children in parts of Africa.

INFECTION

A condition in which the body or part of the body is invaded by a pathogen which, under favourable conditions multiplies and produces injurious affects.

Localised infection is usually accompanied by inflammation.

Spread of infection
By direct contact
During a surgical operation, therefore anything touching the patient should be sterile.
By indirect contact
   Through water – typhoid, cholera
   Through animals – rabies
   Through insects – malaria
   Through the air – droplets transmitting influenza, dust and fluff
Once the organism has gained entry into the body it may spread by various routes:
   Through tissue spaces – cellulitis
   Through the lymphatic vessels – lymphadenitis
   Through the circulatory system – septicaemia
   Passages between two anatomically separate organs – fistula formation
   Capillary deposits – abscesses (bacteria in capillaries – pyaemia), may form abnormal channels to skin surfaces called sinuses.

CROSS INFECTION

Occurs when an infection is transferred from one person to another
General measures to control the spread of infection include
   High standards in personal, departmental and equipment hygiene (see Hygiéne section)
When dealing with an infectious patient ensure that
   Treatment room/X-ray room, equipment and changing cubicles are damp dusted with disinfectant impregnated cloths
   Correct disposal of infected articles is carried out
   Disposable linen is used at all times
   Accessory equipment is covered
   There is correctly functioning air conditioning

Appointment for infectious patients is at the end of the day or when the department is not busy.

BARRIER NURSING

A nursing technique by which patients with an infectious disease are prevented from infecting others. Type of nursing will depend on the individual pathogen.

General measures
If an airborne infection is present the bed must be in a separate room
On the ward it should be placed near to the service area to minimise the risk of transmitting the infection
All articles should be labelled and kept for that patient only
Patient's notes and radiographs to be kept outside the room
Staff attending to the patient wear gowns, masks and gloves whilst in the room
Patient's litter should be burnt
Special instructions to cleaning staff
Warning notices placed in the appropriate area.

Radiography of a barrier nursed patient
2 Radiographers required
   1 handles the patient
   1 handles the equipment
Both wash their hands, put on gown, mask and gloves
Cassette placed in a cover e.g. a pillow case
First radiographer positions the cassette and patient
Second radiographer positions the X-ray tube

After the exposure
First radiographer removes the cassette, holding the cover
Second radiographer removes the cassette from the cover

After the examination
Both wash their hands, remove mask, gloves and gown, and wash their hands again.

REVERSE BARRIER NURSING

This is to prevent any infection being given to the patient e.g.

Patients having received renal transplants
Patients receiving high dose total body irradiation
Any patient with a grossly deficient immune response system
Patients susceptible to diseases – premature babies

Similar procedure as for barrier nursing except that it is the patient and not the staff being protected, therefore any article in direct contact with the patient should be sterile e.g. cassettes should be covered with a sterile cloth. Also staff with colds or infections are not allowed to come into contact with the patient.

INFECTION AND THE RADIOTHERAPY PATIENT

Infection in the tumour area reduces the effectiveness of radiotherapy by impairing the blood supply to the treatment area
This reduces the oxygen tension within the tumour
Anoxic cells are resistant to the effects of radiation
A damaged blood supply hampers the healing process
Permanent damage can lead to necrosis
Carious teeth present a problem when irradiating the mouth – these teeth should be removed before treatment commences as patients who have had dental extractions following treatment may have the problem of impaired healing due to the damage to blood vessels in the bone alveolus
There is also the risk of precipitating maxillary or mandibular necrosis.

Patients with malignant disease are extremely vulnerable to infection for a variety of reasons

Patients may have impairment of their immune response functions
If bone marrow is invaded by malignant disease there will be a reduction in the circulating white cells needed to fight the infection.
Radiotherapy to the bone marrow, spleen and lymph nodes will cause some leucopenia
Most chemotherapy drugs have an adverse effect on the bone marrow, often causing severe leucopenia.

Patients who are greatly at risk from infection are those with blood counts similar to the following:

Total white cell count of less than – $4000/mm^3$ (4×10^9/litre)
Lymphocytes less than   – $1500/mm^3$ ($1 \cdot 5 \times 10^9$/litre)
Neutrophils less than   – $1500/mm^3$ ($1 \cdot 5 \times 10^9$/litre)
Monocytes less than   – $200/mm^3$ (200×10^6/litre)

7

Sterilisation

INTRODUCTION

This chapter deals with the sterilisation procedures which are available for various articles used daily by radiographers.

It is important that inadequately sterilised articles are recognised and discarded, therefore a knowledge of the principles involved in these procedures is necessary.

Student radiographers should be shown how to store sterilised articles and packs and to be able to use stock in the correct order.

Sterilisation is the complete removal of living organisms from an object or body.

Methods available
Moist heat – Autoclaving
                   Boiling (emergency only)
Dry heat – Hot air oven
               Infra red oven
Chemical – Liquid-immersion
                Gases- autoclave
Gamma radiation

MOIST HEAT – AUTOCLAVING

The autoclave (Fig. 7.1)
Has 2 shells – the outer called the jacket
               the inner called the chamber
A hinged access door
Articles are packed loosely in an inner chamber
Chamber is evacuated by a vacuum pump
Steam under pressure is introduced into the jacket and chamber
The steam is at a set temperature and pressure and is introduced for a set time
Steam is removed

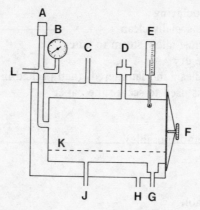

Fig. 7.1 Diagram showing a section through an autoclave
A – Safety valve
B – Pressure gauge
C – Steam inlet to jacket
D – Air inlet to chamber
E – Temperature gauge
F – Safety door
G – Chamber exhaust
H – Jacket exhaust
J – Steam extractor
K – Trivet
L – Steam inlet

Articles are dried in situ
Filtered air is reintroduced.

Tests for efficiency
Pressure and temperature gauges
   Checked for accuracy
Bowie and Dick Test (daily)
   36 towels are folded and packed in a sealed container
   Two pieces of autoclave tape are placed between them (auto-clave tape has brown stripes if sterile, no stripes if not)
   Autoclave is run
   If all the tape has brown stripes and the towels are dry the autoclave is working
Spore test (weekly)
   Non-pathogenic spores (Bacillus stearothermophilus) placed in the autoclave
   Autoclave is run
   The spores are then cultured
   If they fail to germinate, the autoclave is working

Articles for autoclaving
Articles must be socially clean
Paper packets must allow steam to enter
Articles must be dry
Linen must be clean and laundered, then packed in a drum
Autoclave tape is used to secure the paper

Articles suitable
Instruments (non-disposable)
Linen
Dressings

Articles unsuitable
Plastic items
Most disposable items

Typical programme
250 kilopascals (kPa) at 135°C for 3–3½ minutes

After autoclaving
Articles are allowed to dry
Check – Tape is striped
        Seal is not broken
        Packs are dry

MOIST HEAT – BOILING (emergency use only)

The steriliser
Metal container with a lid
Large enough to hold the article and water
Usually electrically heated

Use of the steriliser
Articles packed loosely into the steriliser
Articles must be below the water level
The lid is placed on the steriliser
The water is brought to a 'full rolling boil'
Articles are then boiled for 5 minutes
N.B. If an additional article is added, the water must be brought back to the boil and timing recommenced.
Once boiled the articles are handled with sterile cheatle forceps
Articles are cooled before use

Articles suitable
Metal instruments and utensils
Glass syringes
Needles
Rubber catheters

Articles unsuitable
Plastic tubing (except P.V.C.)
Delicate instruments, endoscopes, laryngoscopes etc.

Disadvantages
No standardisation
Time consuming
Easily contaminated
No check on the sterility of the articles

Cheatle forceps (Fig. 7.2)
Long handled forceps
Kept in a jar of disinfectant
2 pairs required
Always hold with points down to prevent contamination of the forceps
Do not allow them to touch unsterile objects

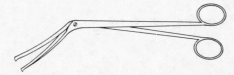

Fig 7.2 Cheatle forceps

DRY HEAT

Hot air oven
Socially clean articles placed in the oven
Articles must not be tightly packed

Typical programme
160°C for 1 hour

Articles suitable
Hardened delicate glasswear

Delicate instruments
All glass syringes

Articles unsuitable
Rubber
Plastic

GAMMA RADIATION

Unit
Socially clean articles placed on a moving conveyor belt
Radiation source is of short wavelength

Typical dosage
2.5×10^6 centigrays (cGy)

Sterile packs
Have a red dot if sterile
Or are marked gamma ray sterilised

Articles suitable
Those which would be damaged by heat
Plastic catheters
Knife holders
Disposable instruments, gloves etc.

CHEMICAL

Principles
Articles – must be socially clean
          must be submerged for the required length of time
Chemical – either in solution or gaseous
          must be sufficiently strong
          more effective hot than cold
Container – must be sterile
          can be an autoclave

Types of chemical
Bacteriocidal – agent kills bacteria
Bacteriostatic – agent inhibits growth of bacteria
Germicidal – agent which kills germs
Antiseptic – inhibits the growth of bacteria

Chemical gas

Ethylene oxide – used in an autoclave at 55°C and 220 kilopascals
for 3 hours
Suitable for most plastics

Liquid disinfectants

Quaternary ammonium compounds – skin antiseptics
Iodines – germicidal
Alcohols – antiseptic
Formaldehyde – powerful germicide

CENTRAL STERILE SUPPLY DEPARTMENT (C.S.S.D.)

Advantages

Standardisation of pack contents
Packs available at short notice
Labour saving
Less handling of articles
Packs are available for specific procedures

Disadvantages

Risk of cross infection
Large stock of articles required
Transportation between the unit and department may be difficult

Presentation

Packs double wrapped with water repellent paper
Drums and boxes are used

Use of C.S.S.D. packs

A record book is used when ordering packs
Store packs in a cool, dry place
Packs used in strict rotation
Shelf life 7–12 days unless they have a plastic cover
Check
  Correct pack
  Tape is striped
  Seal is not broken
  Pack is dry
Open outer pack
Shake the contents onto a sterile surface
Open contents, touching the outside cover only
After use, clean and return articles.

8

Instruments and dressings

INTRODUCTION

This section is intended as an introduction to some of the instruments and dressings which the student radiographer may come across during the training period.

Although radiographers will not have direct responsibility for the use of some of the instruments, it is desirable for them to understand how the instruments are used.

It is usual for students to be taught about instruments and dressings under clinical supervision, which should enable the students to develop a competent practical technique when called upon to assist in any procedures involving the use of instruments and dressings.

Biopsy forceps (Fig. 8.1)
Long metal forceps with crocodile action of the end blades, used for taking tissue samples from narrow passages e.g. the throat. They operate with a scissor action. Must be sterilised before use.

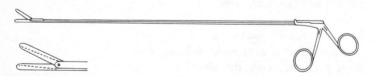

Fig. 8.1 Biopsy forceps

Brook airway (Fig. 8.2)
Used for expired air ventilation to avoid direct contact with the patient. The mouth guard provides a seal over the patient's mouth. Patient's exhaled air escapes through an exhaust port. Socially clean before use.

Catheters (excluding urinary catheters):
Tubing of either rubber or plastic for the introduction of substances into the body. Sterilise before use.

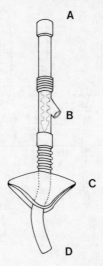

Fig. 8.2 Brook/Airway
A – Operator's mouth piece
B – Exit port for patient's exhaled air
C – Mouth guard
D – Patient's mouth piece

Cannula (Fig. 8.3)

An artificial tube inserted into body cavities, part of the tube may be expanded to reduce leakage. Sterilise before use.

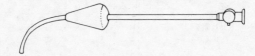

Fig. 8.3 Cannula

Cervical dilator (Fig. 8.4)

Metal instrument used to dilate the cervix e.g. prior to the insertion of radioactive caesium or prior to hysterosalpingography. Sterilise before use.

Chiba needle (Fig. 8.5)

A 15 cm long, thin, stainless steel needle used to inject a contrast agent directly into an intrahepatic duct during percutaneous cholangiography. Sterilise before use.

Clinical thermometer

Used for taking the patient's temperature, may be of oral, rectal or low temperature type. Sterilise before use.

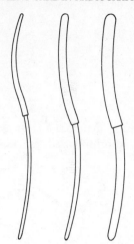

Fig. 8.4 Cervical dilators

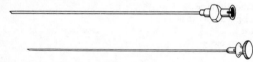

Fig. 8.5 Chiba needle

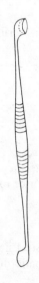

Fig. 8.6 Curette

Curette (Fig. 8.6)

A double, spoon ended, instrument for reducing or excising a basal cell carcinoma. Sterilise before use.

Drip infusion sets
Consist of a bottle, tubing and a needle. Used for introducing a substance into a patient over a long period of time. e.g. Infusion cholangiography, chemotherapy drugs. Sterile procedure – apart from rectal infusion.

Endotracheal tube
Passed down the trachea to maintain a clear airway, used in anaesthetics and may be cuffed or uncuffed. Sterilise before use.

Forceps
Cheatle forceps. Long handled forceps, usually metal, used for removing sterile instruments out of solution. Must always be held with the points down. Sterilise before use.

Dissecting forceps. (Fig. 8.7) Used for picking up 'light' articles (heavy articles turn the blades out of true). Used during biopsies and for performing sterile dressings using no-touch technique. Sterilise before use.

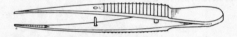

Fig. 8.7   Dissecting forceps – non toothed

Sponge holding forceps. (Fig. 8.8) Rounded ends, used for holding swabs when cleaning a patient e.g. prior to femoral arteriography or hysterosalpingography. Sterilise before use.

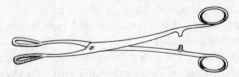

Fig. 8.8   Sponge holding forceps

Tissue forceps. (Fig. 8.9) Pointed ends which can be clipped together, used for holding the skin. Sterilise before use.

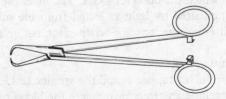

Fig. 8.9   Tissue forceps

Gallipots

Either plastic or tin foil (disposable) or metal (reusable) bowls used to hold solutions. Sterilise before use.

Laryngeal mirror (Fig. 8.10)

Small mirror on a metal rod, used for examining the oral cavity and during indirect laryngoscopies. Socially clean before use.

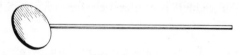

Fig. 8.10   Laryngeal mirror

Laryngoscope

An instrument used to visually inspect the larynx to see if there is any obstruction present and can be used to take tissue samples if necessary. Sterilise before use.

Needles

Pointed narrow tubes for the introduction of substances, by subcutaneous, intramuscular or intravenous means, or to aspirate fluid. Usually disposable. The coloured, plastic fitting denotes the size. Sterilise before use.

Lumbar puncture needle. Long needle used for performing a lumbar puncture, for the removal of cerebrospinal fluid or the introduction of a contrast agent. Sterilise before use.

Drawing up needle. Long, wide ended needle used for filling syringes. Sterilise before use.

Sialography needle. Used for injecting contrast agents into the salivary glands. Metal, with an expanded area to prevent the agent from spilling out of the gland. Sterilise before use.

Ophthalmoscope

Instrument for examining the eye. Consists of a mirror with a hole in it, through which the observer looks. The inner aspect of the eye (retina) is illuminated by light reflected from the mirror. Can be fitted with different size lenses. Socially clean before use.

Pneumatic cuff

Rubber /fabric cuff, wrapped round the arm/leg and expanded with air. Used to occlude an artery or measure the blood pressure. Maximum time for which it should be inflated on the patient's limb is 10 minutes or gangrene may result. Socially clean before use.

Receiver
Large metal bowl used to receive dirty swabs and instruments usually during a sterile procedure. Socially clean before use.

Seldinger trocar and cannula (Fig. 8.11)
Used for the introduction of a guide wire/catheter into an artery.

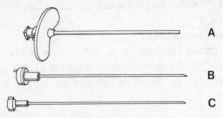

Fig. 8.11 Seldinger trocar and cannula
A – Cannula
B – Trocar
C – Stillette

Trocar has a pointed end, and fits inside the cannula (more than one trocar may be required if a large cannula is used). Both are introduced, the trocar is removed and the guide wire is inserted through the cannula. The catheter is then fed over the guide wire. Can be used to insert a cannula to drain fluid from a cavity. Sterilise before use.

Scalpel blades
Usually disposable metal blade (and plastic holder) used in surgery for opening the skin surface. Sterilise before use.

Sphygmomanometer
Instrument for measuring the blood pressure. Socially clean before use.

Surgical masks
Cloth/paper and polythene/paper masks which cover the nose and mouth. Paper masks worn for a maximum of 10 minutes, must be changed if become moist.

Swabs
Pieces of gauze or paper material for cleaning, packing superficial wounds. Sterilise before use.

Filamented swabs – have a radiopaque strip. Used in theatre for internal swabbing as the swab can be traced radiographically if lost. Sterilise before use.

Syringes

Either plastic (disposable) or glass and metal (reusable) have graduated markings on the side and an end fitting. Sterilise before use.

Higginson's syringe – rubber syringe with a balloon and a one way valve. Used for pumping air e.g. into the rectum during a barium enema. Socially clean before use.

Uterine sound (Fig. 8.12)

Long, blunt ended, curved instrument with a scale on the side. Used for assessing the length and direction of the uterus prior to hysterosalpingography. Sterilise before use.

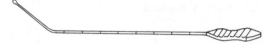

Fig. 8.12   Uterine sound

Vaginal speculum (Fig. 8.13)

Metal or plastic instrument inserted into the vagina to enable the examination of the cervix and uterus and to allow the introduction of instruments. Sterilise before use.

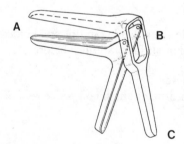

Fig. 8.13   Vaginal speculum
A – Inserted into the vagina
B – For the introduction of instruments
C – Handles

Victoria enema ring

Circular, rubber disc, the rim of which can be inflated with air, used during barium enema examinations to contain the barium in the event of involuntary defaecation. Socially clean before use.

Vomit bowls
Metal/plastic/paper bowls with a long handle used to receive vomit. Socially clean before use.

9

Patient preparation — Diagnostic

INTRODUCTION

Every patient who enters an X-ray department will require some form of preparation. It is important that the student radiographer understands that such routine checks such as the patient's full name and address must be carried out carefully or a situation may occur which leads to the wrong patient being radiographed.

The importance of correct abdominal preparation cannot be overemphasized as faecal matter may obscure small detail in the abdomen such as renal calculi.

A chart at the end of the chapter outlines the patient preparation before and after specific examinations. The preparation may vary from department to department because of individual preference and therefore example preparations only are given.

Preparation may take place immediately prior to a radiographic examination or may extend over several days.

THE 10 DAY RULE

To prevent the unnecessary irradiation of an early fetus the 10 day rule has been devised. Therefore for examination of the abdomen, pelvis or hips (which are considered by the referring Doctor to be non-urgent) any woman of childbearing age is asked to complete an L.M.P. form. The form asks for the date of the first day of the last menstrual period (L.M.P.) and usually gives a brief explanation of the 10 day rule.

Examinations of the pelvic region may only take place within the first 10 days, from the commencement of the menstrual period.

OUT PATIENT PREPARATION

The patient should be given written details of:
Time and date of the examination

A simple explanation of the examination
Full details of any preparation required
Approximate length of time of the examination
Name of the hospital and department
Hospital telephone number and department extension
N.B. The 10 day rule should be considered when booking the appointment with a request that the patient should notify the department if there is any change in the menstrual cycle.

IN PATIENT PREPARATION

The information should be sent to the Ward Sister/Charge nurse of the ward concerned.
Name and record number of the patient
Date and time of the examination
Nature of the examination
Details of any preparation required

GENERAL PREPARATION

Ask the patient his/her name and check with the request form
Check the patient's:
    address
    age
    occupation
    ward (if applicable)
    L.M.P. (if applicable)
Ask if the patient has been radiographed before, if so where and when
Ask if they have followed any instructions which may have been given previously
Check if any adverse effects have occured following the ingestion of any tablets/medicines, or earlier X-ray examinations
Give a full explanation of any clothing which has to be removed
Ensure clean gown and dressing gown are available

PREPARATION FOR ABDOMINAL EXAMINATIONS

It is necessary to remove intestinal gas and faeces which may obscure visualisation of small detail e.g. renal calculi, gall stones.

FLATULENCE

This is the presence of excessive gas in the gastro-intestinal tract.

Causes

Nervous stress – Causing muscle spasm. Air swallowing (aerophagy)
Diet – High carbohydrate intake. High fat intake
Immobility – Patient may be bedridden
Patient may have a limited range of movement
Preparation – The over-use of aperients
Inadequate explanation/reassurance
Drugs/drinks – Carbonated drinks

Prevention

Reassurance – Prevents the patient from worrying
Recommend no smoking, to prevent aerophagy (N.B. this may cause gas if the patient becomes anxious without cigarettes)
Low residue diet – e.g. mince, mashed vegetables, fish, milk based foods
Activity – Encourage movement/exercise
Aperients – Ensure the recommended dose is not exceeded
(Note list of contraindications under aperients)

Elimination

Drugs
   e.g. Buscopan two, 10 mg tablets
   Polycrol 1 or 2 tablets
          5–10 ml fluid
Charcoal biscuits/burnt toast
   Prescribed because charcoal absorbs gas
Flatus tube
   Thick rectal tube with an expanded end opening
   Tube connected to a funnel
   Rounded end of tube lubricated and inserted into the rectum
   Funnel placed under water so that the gas can be seen escaping

FAECES

Waste products of digestion

Elimination

Aperients. Induce gentle peristaltic action of the bowel causing defaecation.
N.B. Large doses can cause pain, spasm, diarrhoea, flatulence.
   Diet. A laxative effect can be obtained by a diet that contains sufficient roughage e.g. fruits, vegetables

Lubricants. These lubricate the colon wall and ease the passage of softened faecal matter e.g. Paraffin emulsion, castor oil.

Bulk producing. The contents retain water and mix with the intestinal contents to form a soft mass which encourages peristalsis e.g. Prepacol

Colonic activators. Stimulate colonic peristalsis e.g. X Prep, Dulcolax, Dulcolax suppositories.

Contraindications for the use of aperients
Haemorrhage/obstruction of the alimentary tract
Ulcerative colitis
Diverticulosis/diverticulitis
Diarrhoea
Megacolon
Young children

Enematic and colonic lavage

Enema
Fluid is introduced into the colon per rectum, or via a colostomy
    To remove faecal matter from the bowel
    To replace lost body fluids
    To administer drugs
To remove faecal matter
Fluids used:
    Soap and water (enema saponis)
    Olive oil
    Glycerine
Trolley setting:
    Lubricant on a swab
    Disposable towel
    Container for the solution
    Catheter/tubing
    Clips
    Bedpan/commode
Procedure:
    Screens placed round the patient
    Patient lies on their left side, hips and knees flexed
    Protective sheet is placed under the patient
    Air is expelled from the funnel and catheter by running through some liquid and clamping off the tubing
    Catheter is lubricated and inserted into the rectum
    Approximately 1 litre of solution is administered, at a temperature of 5°C

Catheter is removed
Patient is asked to retain the enema for 3 minutes
Patient is placed on a bedpan and the bowel contents are evacuated
Patient is cleaned and made comfortable

Colonic lavage
Performed to empty the bowel prior to examination or operation.
Fluid used:
    Water
Trolley setting:
    See Enema
Procedure:
    Patient lies on their left side, hips and knees flexed
    Catheter inserted into the rectum
    Solution is administered
    Solution is 'run out' through the catheter
    Process continues until clear fluid returns

Diet modification
Patient may be requested to have nothing to eat or drink prior to the examination e.g. if a general anaesthetic is required or in opaque meals (e.g. barium).
    Patient follows a low residue diet for 48 hours prior e.g. Minced meat, fish etc. avoiding green vegetables, cereals, whole meal bread, fatty foods.
    Patient avoids gas forming foods e.g. parsnips, peas, beans, effervescent drinks and starchy foods.

Patients who require special care

Diabetic patients
Medical consultation prior to diet modification
Given laxatives only
Always placed first on a list
If the patient has to starve, told to omit insulin and bring food and insulin with him

Children
No abdominal preparation required

Bed patients
Encouraged to sit up or if possible walk around to avoid flatulence.

NURSING CARE BEFORE AND AFTER SPECIFIC EXAMINATIONS

Before all examinations it is essential that

The patient's identity is checked

They are given a full explanation of the procedure

They are reassured

The date of the last menstrual period is checked (if appropriate)

Emergency drugs are available when iodine based contrast agents are used

Examination	Definition	Patient preparation before the examination	Patient care after the examination
Angiography (general)	Demonstration of the circulatory system by the injection of an iodine based contrast agent into an artery	Abdominal preparation may be required. Consent form signed. Premedication given. Nothing by mouth 5 hours prior. Warned of metallic taste following injection of the contrast agent	Observe injection site for haematoma following digital pressure. Spray injection site with plastic skin dressing. Pulse and blood pressure taken every 30 minutes for 4 hours. Then every 4 hours for 24 hours
Carotid angiography	Demonstration of the brain circulation by direct injection into the carotid artery or via a catheter in the femoral artery, which is passed to the carotid artery	See angiography (general). Shave groin if femoral catheter used	See angiography (general)
Femoral arteriography	Direct injection into a palpable artery in the leg (usually femoral)	See angiography (general)	See angiography (general)

Examination	Definition	Patient preparation before the examination	Patient care after the examination
Translumbar aortography	Investigation of the aorta and major branches by direct injection into the abdominal aorta	See angiography (general) Shave as necessary	See angiography (general)
Arch aortography	Investigation of the aorta and major branches by femoral or axillary catheterization	See angiography (general) Shave as necessary (groin or axilla)	See angiography (general)
Renal arteriography	Investigation of the renal areas by catheterization of the femoral artery	See angiography (general) Micturate prior to the examination Shave groin	See angiography (general)
Angiocardiography (cardiac catheterization)	Demonstration of the heart and great vessels by brachial or femoral catheterization	See angiography (general) Shave as neccesary	See angiography (general)
Arthrography (e.g. knee)	Investigation of joint anatomy following the injection of air or an iodine based contrast agent into the joint capsule	Preliminary films taken Knee shaved Transport home arranged	Rest with limb elevated for 12 hours
Opaque meal e.g. Barium	Examination of the stomach by the ingestion of a radiopaque contrast agent	Abdominal preparation Nothing by mouth 8 hours prior Warn of possible follow through examination	Ensure mouth is clean Warn of possible constipation Inform the patient that he can return to normal diet

Opaque swallow e.g. Barium	Examination of the oesophagus by the ingestion of a radiopaque contrast agent	As for a Barium meal	As for a Barium meal
Opaque enema e.g. Barium	Examination of the colon by the introduction of a radiopaque contrast agent or a radiopaque and a radiolucent contrast agent, via a rectal catheter or a colostomy	Abdominal preparation Colonic lavage (may be required) Asked to retain the contrast agent Informed of the evacuation stage Ensure toilet facilities are available	Warn of possible constipation Ensure clean and comfortable Provide a fresh bag for colostomy patients
Bronchography	Investigation of the bronchial tree following the introduction of contrast agent via the trachea	Postural drainage for 3 days prior Requested not to cough during the procedure Nothing by mouth for 5 hours prior Light premedication given Local anaesthetic may be required	Allowed to cough Nothing by mouth for 3 hours – warn of the danger of inhaling food or drink Postural drainage may be required
Oral cholecystography	Investigation of the biliary tract by the ingestion of a contrast agent	Preliminary film taken Abdominal preparation Fat free diet 12 hours prior Contrast agent taken 12 hours prior Then nothing by mouth except fat free fluids	Return to normal diet

Examination	Definition	Patient preparation before the examination	Patient care after the examination
Endoscopic retrograde choledocho – pancreatography (E.R.C.P.)	Investigation of the pancreatic and biliary systems. The contrast agent is injected into the papilla of Vater via a fibre-optic endoscope	Nothing by mouth for 5 hours prior Premedication given Recent radiographs of the biliary tract area should be available Pharynx is anesthetised Endoscope is introduced	Nothing by mouth for 2 hours Serum amylase level is checked the following day (any rise in the level is indicative of pancreatitis)
Intravenous cholangiography	Investigation of the biliary tract by injection of a radiopaque contrast agent (undertaken when oral cholecystography has failed)	As for oral cholecystography but contrast agent given on the day of the examination Check for history of allergy Arm prepared for an intravenous injection	Return to normal diet
Infusion cholangiography	As above but contrast agent infused	As above	Return to normal diet
Dacryocystography	Investigation of the lacrimal system following the direct injection of an iodine based contrast agent	Local anaesthetic required	Eye covered until the 'blinking' action returns
Air encephalography	Investigation of the ventricles of the brain following the introduction of air via a lumbar puncture	Skull and chest radiographed Nothing by mouth for 5 hours prior Consent form signed Micturate prior to the examination Premedication given	Bed rest for 24 hours Pulse and blood pressure recorded every 15 minutes for 4 hours then temperature, pulse, respiration, blood pressure recorded every 4 hours for 24 hours

Ventriculography	Investigation of the ventricles of the brain by the direct injection of air into the ventricles via a burr hole, in the skull vault	See air encephalography But catheter introduced into the ventricles under general anaesthetic, air is then injected and films taken when the patient recovers	See air encephalography
Excretion urography (intravenous pyelography I.V.P.)	Investigation of the kidneys, ureters and bladder following injection of an iodine based contrast agent	Abdominal preparation Fluid may be restricted for 12 hours prior Check for history of allergies Patient asked to micturate prior to examination	Non-specific
Lymphography	Investigation of the lymphatic system following a direct injection of the contrast agent into a lymphatic vessel of the foot	If oedema of the leg, admitted for several days Chest X-Ray Abdominal preparation Dorsum of foot shaved Warn patient and relatives of change in skin colour Warn patient of change in urine colour and vision will have blue/green haze Empty bladder prior to examination	Pressure bandages applied to foot Inform the patient that further films may be required Keep foot dry because of sutures in situ
Myelography	Investigation of the spinal canal following the injection of air or myodil via a lumbar puncture	Recent radiographic examination of the spine Nothing by mouth for 5 hours prior to examination The contrast agent may be introduced on the ward	Pulse and blood pressure every 30 minutes for 4 hours Patient kept flat for 24 hours

Examination	Definition	Patient preparation before the examination	Patient care after the examination
Radiculography	As for myelography but a water soluble contrast agent is used	See myelography	Trunk and head *raised* for 8 hours Bed rest 24 hours Pulse and blood pressure every, 30 minutes for 4 hours
Retrograde pyelograph	Performed when an I.V.P. has failed Introduction of a catheter into the renal pelvis via the urethra and bladder to introduce an iodine based contrast agent	Abdominal preparation Consent form signed Warned not to remove the catheter Starvation for 4 hours prior Premedication given General anaesthetic	4 hourly observations of temperature, pulse and respiration for 24 hours Return to normal diet
Cystography	The introduction of a radiopaque contrast agent into the bladder via a catheter	Empty bladder Requested to retain the contrast agent Toilet facilities available Nervous patients may require a sedative	May be given Sulphonamides for 4 days following to counteract infection
Male urethro-graphy	Investigation of the male urethra following the introduction of an iodine based contrast agent	Full explanation given Micturate prior to the examination Local anaesthetic given	Warned that haematuria may occur Sulphonamides may be prescribed

Hysterosalpingography	Investigation of the uterus and uterine tubes following cannulation of the cervix	Examination takes place after menstruation and within the 10 days of the 10 day rule Empty bladder prior to the examination Premedication/general anaesthetic may be required Recovery room prepared	Patient rests if necessary Warned of possible haemorrhage
Sialography	Investigation of the salivary glands following the direct injection of an iodine based contrast agent	Preliminary films required Patient removes false teeth Patient is given a lemon to suck to open the ampulla of the duct	Mouth wash is given
Peripheral venography	Investigation of the venous system of a limb following direct injection of an iodine based contrast agent into a vein	Nothing by mouth for 5 hours prior to the examination Micturate prior to the examination Premedication given	When premedication has worn off, encourage to walk about
Portal venography	Investigation of the portal system following the direct injection of an iodine based contrast agent into the spleen	Abdominal preparation Micturate prior to examination Premedication given Nothing by mouth for 5 hours prior	Bed rest for 5 hours Pulse and blood pressure every 15 minutes for 4 hours Temperature, pulse, respiration, blood pressure every 4 hours for 24 hours Analgesics may be required

Example of a typical abdominal preparation
Low residue diet 48 hours prior
Avoid gas forming foods 48 hours prior
Laxative given 36 and 12 hours prior to the examination.

PATIENT PREPARATION FOR OTHER IMAGING TECHNIQUES

ULTRASOUND

General preparation
Check identity of the patient
Give explanation and reassurance
Removal of clothing from the area of interest
Mineral oil or ultrasonic gel spread over the area to be examined
Change the sheets between patients

Preparation for specific examinations

Abdomen
Problem of bowel gas as this reflects ultrasonic waves
Abdominal preparation may be required
Practice breathing techniques
Should be no barium sulphate present in the patient as this prevents the passage of ultrasonic waves

Gall bladder
Fat free diet prior to the examination – to ensure the gall bladder is full of bile
If performed during cholecystography – should be prior to the fatty meal

Obstetrics and gynaecology
Full urinary bladder required — displaces bowel gas in early pregnancy and gives a 'window' to view the uterus and lifts the fetal head out of the pelvis later in pregnancy
Liaison with the ante natal clinic as patients are often requested to give a urine sample — ultrasound should be done first
Clinical history should be available
Patient may feel faint due to pressure of the fetus on the inferior vena cava. If this occurs turn the patient onto the side to relieve pressure.

Biopsy and aspiration techniques
Signed consent form required
Previous radiographs and case notes required
Aseptic technique
Amniocentesis – patient should rest following the examination

RADIONUCLIDE IMAGING

General preparation
Check the identity of the patient
Give an explanation and reassure the patient 10 day rule is observed
Large opacities e.g. breast prosthesis, buckles, medallions should be removed
Recent radiograph of the area required
   e.g. Brain scans   – skull radiographs
         Renogram patients – radiograph of the kidneys

Other considerations

Radioactivity
After the injection, patients should not sit near pregnant women because of the radiation hazard
Nursing mothers should not breast feed for 48 hours as their milk may be contaminated

Contamination
Urine and vomit disposed of down the toilet
Linen stored in marked, plastic bags which allows for the various decay rates of the isotopes used

Emptying bladder
Done prior to bone scans – the radiopharmaceutical is excreted via the kidney, and bladder uptake may obscure the bony pelvis

Diet
Renogram examinations – may require fluid intake restriction
Gastric emptying and thyroid uptakes – patient starved overnight

Drugs
Potassium perchlorate is given to prevent the thyroid gland from absorbing the isotope in certain examinations e.g. brain scans

Certain thyroid medications are withdrawn prior to thyroid uptake examinations

Examinations involving iodine based contrast agents should be delayed until after scanning or concentration will not take place during scanning

Provided that the patient is not on oral iron, an intra muscular injection of Jectofer, 100mg, may be given 2 hours prior to the administration of the radionuclide gallium (to limit the amount of gallium absorbed by the wall of the intestine). The scan is performed 24 hours later

Bowel preparation

Laxatives may be required prior to the administration of the radionuclide gallium. The radionuclide is injected 2 days previously and the laxative is given the day before scanning, this clears the bowel of faecal matter.

COMPUTERISED TOMOGRAPHY

General preparation

Check the identity of the patient
Give an explanation and reassure the patient
Remove opacities from the area of the examination

Preparation for specific examinations

Brain scans

Large bandages may have to be removed as they make packing of the head difficult
Anaesthetic may be required
Premedication for young children

Whole body scans

Abdominal preparation may be required
Abdomen should be free from contrast agents e.g. barium sulphate
Propantheline: 30–45mg intra muscular, 10 minutes prior to eliminate bowel movement
Arrows placed on bony landmarks e.g. xiphisternum, lower costal margin
Gastrografin may be given to demonstrate the colon but calcium sulphate will be required orally 2–3 days prior
Solubiloptin may be added to the gastrografin to demonstrate the gall bladder

Intravenous contrast agents can be administered to demonstrate the circulatory system and therefore a check on patient allergies should be made

NUCLEAR MAGNETIC RESONANCE
Research is now being undertaken on nuclear magnetic resonance, and clinical studies are taking place.

General preparation
Check the identity of the patient
Give explanation and reassure the patient
Remove opacities from the area of the examination
Check the patient does not have a pacemaker – as this will be affected by the magnetic field
Check the patient does not have a history of epilepsy – the magnetic field may cause a fit
Check the patient does not have a history of myocardial infarction

Specific preparation
Will probably be similar to that of computerised tomography except that as blood flow can be demonstrated without the use of contrast agents these will probably not be required.

10

Patient preparation — Radiotherapy Care of radiation reactions

INTRODUCTION

Advancing radiation treatment techniques are designed to spare normal tissue wherever possible, whilst delivering a high tumour dose to a prescribed area.

Unfortunately, some irradiation of normal cells is unavoidable and these produce 'side effects'.

To alleviate the worries caused to the patients by these side effects, the radiotherapy team of radiographers, radiotherapists and nursing staff should be able to give a clear explanation to these patients and be able to minimise the side effects with a high standard of treatment and nursing care.

REACTIONS IN SPECIFIC SITES

Treatment with megavoltage radiation gives some degree of protection to the skin as the maximum dose occurs at a depth below the surface. Skin tumours e.g. basal cell carcinoma, squamous cell carcinoma, and patients requiring postoperative irradiation on a mastectomy scar, will be requiring doses of radiation either on machines with a kVp range of 110 kVp – 250 kVp, or megavoltage machines with 'build up' material placed on the patient's scar region. These patients will experience very brisk skin reactions. Fair and auburn haired people tolerate radiation less well than dark haired/skinned people.

STAGES OF ACUTE SKIN REACTIONS

First degree following a single dose to the skin of 750 – 1000 cGy
Erythema – reddening of the skin, caused by congestion of the blood vessels (temporary)

Second degree following a single dose of the skin of 1000–1500 cGy

Bright erythema
Epilation
Arrest of sweat production (may be permanent)
Erythema starts to disappear when basal cells start to regenerate
Peeling off of extra dead cells from the surface – dry desquamation

Third degree following a single radiation dose to the skin of
1500–2000 cGy
   3250 cGy in 5 treatments over 1 week
   5000 cGy in 20 treatments over 4 weeks
Deep erythema
Loss of epithelial cell structure
Release of intra/extra cellular fluid – moist desquamation, dries
with scab formation
Permanent epilation
Destruction of sweat glands
All of the above are 'normal' reactions.

Fourth degree
Radiation necrosis – can be caused by radiation overdosage
Breakdown of epidermis and dermis
Destruction of blood vessels
Damage to sensory nerve endings therefore necrotic area very
painful
Healing delayed or nonexistent

LATE CHANGES FOLLOWING ACUTE SKIN REACTIONS

Pigmentation
Due to increased synthesis of melanin
Increased number of melanocytes
Migration of melanocytes within the epidermis

Telangiectasia
Dilatation of terminal capillaries to compensate for artery impairment around the irradiated area. (Can occur anywhere in the body)

Ischaemia
Destruction of blood vessels leading to a reduced blood supply to
the skin (and other organs)
Makes subsequent healing in the area difficult

Total loss of blood supply leads to necrosis
The irradiated skin will always be more susceptible to damage and the patient must be told of care needed for this area.

No exposure to intense sunlight, wind or cold
Prevent the area from receiving friction/irritants which could precipitate skin breakdown.

CARE OF THE PATIENT FOLLOWING RADIOTHERAPY

Explain the anticipated reaction
Treatment area kept free from friction e.g.

No rubbing the skin
No shaving
No tight clothing around the treatment area.

During the treatment period the area may be dusted with a light chalk powder which often helps to keep the skin more comfortable against the patient's clothing. Contraindicated are powders containing metallic oxides as the presence of these metals would create a characteristic radiation which would add to the skin dose
Any dressing within the treatment area should be kept in place by Netalast bandage or a nonmetallic tape such as Micropore tape.
Watch for a reaction from an exit dose on megavoltage units
For a skin reaction proceeding to moist desquamation

Discontinue the powdering
Dressings to cover the area when in a public place to help prevent infecting the area
Use of an antibiotic cream or spray e.g. Graneodin

This reaction may be seen on patients on megavoltage units having a radical beam directed treatment over a period of five to six weeks for a fairly superficial tumour e.g. carcinoma of the anterior section of the vocal cord. A tissue equivalent wax is placed on the beam direction shell which will then contain the build-up region thereby bringing the maximum dose to the skin surface.
N.B. There should be frequent medical consultations for patients with brisk skin reactions.

NURSING CARE FOR EXTREME REACTIONS TO RADIOTHERAPY

An old fashioned but effective remedy

Gauze soaked in a 1 per cent aqueous gentian violet solution
Placed on reaction area

Kept in place, resoaked daily with the solution for one week
Allowed to dry
Gauze will gradually separate off, leaving the healed skin underneath.
Patients are usually admitted to hospital for this treatment.
Contraindicated is the use of any creams which exclude the air (air is important in the healing process) e.g. white petroleum jelly.

REACTIONS IN THE ORAL CAVITY

Arising following irradiation of the oral cavity
High dose radiotherapy to an oral tumour treating to a tumour dose (T.D.) of 6000 cGy in 25 treatments over 5 weeks
Following irradiation of neck and thorax for a lymphoma (Mantle technique)
T.D. 3500 cGy in 20 treatments over 4 weeks
The oral cavity and the pharynx are lined with mucous membrane which is highly sensitive to radiation.

1st stage
Inflammation of the lining
Goblet cells cease to function
Mouth becomes sore and dry

2nd stage
Formation of a protective white membrane – from fluid released from damaged cells
Fluid mixes with dead surface cells

3rd stage
Membrane adheres to underlying damaged tissue, repair begins
Radiation effects on the salivary glands adds to the dryness
Saliva contains a bacteriostatic agent which helps prevent the mouth from becoming infected

Care of the patient
Before radiotherapy commences all patients, with their own teeth, should have them inspected. Any carious teeth should be removed before treatment
Good dental and oral hygiene should be encouraged
Radiotherapy may precipitate dental decay due to
Reduction in the blood supply to the teeth
Exposure of the tooth root if the radiation causes gum shrinkage

Risk of infection due to impairment of the salivary glands
Some degree of protection can be afforded by bridging the teeth
with a protective cap during the treatment and reaction period.

Patients suffering from dysphagia
Benzocaine mucilage before meals is an effective analgesic.
Use of frequent mouthwashes e.g. glycerin and thymol
Gentle teeth cleaning
Antiseptic mouthwashes may be substituted if infection is present
e.g. Betadine (an iodine based antiseptic)
Fungal infections can be prevented by a mouthwash e.g. contain-
ing Nystatin
Food may be liquidised, nothing too hot or spicy
Alcoholic spirits should be avoided
Anorexia will be a problem because of the soreness and lack of
taste due to impairment of the taste buds.

REACTIONS OF THE BOWEL

The most sensitive area of the bowel to radiation is the small in-
testine
Consists of a lining of columnar epithelium
Goblet cells are scattered among the epithelial cells
Surface is covered by millions of projections called villi which
greatly increase the surface area
The generative cells for epithelial replacement are found at the
base of the villi – the crypts.

Crypts
Radiation causes the cells to swell up and disintegrate
Debris collects in them.

Villi
Shorten because of lack of replacement cells
Total destruction of a large area of intestinal villi would lead to
death of the patient
Radiation doses for malignant disease in the abdomen and pelvis
are not sufficient to cause total and irreversible damage, villi re-
generation quickly returns

Diarrhoea
May occur hours after commencement of treatment indicating the

speed with which the absorbing properties of the bowel are affected.

Care of the patient
The patient should be warned that the reactions are normal.

For the treatment of the diarrhoea
Attention to diet – resist all foods which loosen the stools
High fluid intake – In patients will have a fluid balance chart
Troublesome diarrhoea responds to
   Codeine phosphate 30 mg 3 times daily
   Imodium 2 mg 3 times daily

Tenesmus
Patient may complain of severe spasmodic abdominal cramps (tenesmus) this arises due to acute inflammation in the treatment area
Peristalsis is affected leading to constipation above the inflammed area
Pethidine will relieve the pain – 50 mg orally
Peristalsis will be helped with 10 ml pethidine in hot water
It is expected that patients experiencing acute bowel reactions will be nursed on the radiotherapy ward

EPILATION

This is loss of hair – temporary below a skin dose causing
   moist desquamation
   permanent at a skin dose causing moist desquamation
Radiotherapy. Epilation only occurs within the treatment and exit dose areas.
Chemotherapy. Epilation caused by some drugs is a general effect Occurs because of the effect on the regenerating cells of the hair in the hair bulb, if there is total destruction of these cells permanent epilation will result.
Psychologically epilation is extremely damaging for many patients. If patients are expected to have total hair loss over a period of time, they should be referred to the NHS wig specialist before the hair loss occurs

RADIATION EFFECTS ON THE BONE MARROW

Bone marrow is highly sensitive to radiation

Red bone marrow
Produces the blood cells
Large field irradiation significantly affects blood cell production
In adult life red bone marrow is found in the
    sternum
    iliac crests
    skull
    upper end of humeri
    upper end of femori
    scapulae
    clavicles
    vertebrae

Blood counts
A drop in peripheral platelet and white cell counts may be noticeable following only a few treatment sessions.
White cells have a relatively short life span – average 7 days.
Red cells with a life span of 120 days are not affected so rapidly.
Patients with falling blood counts should be sent for regular blood counts, daily blood counts may be required.

Care of the patient

Leucopenia – reduced white cell count. Do not treat patient with a white blood count below 2000/mm^3 (2.0 × 10^9/litre) – this leads to a reduced ability to cope with infections.

Patients should be warned of the risks of going to public places like theatres, should avoid people with diagnosed infections and should report any ill health or temperature rise immediately.

Patients contracting infections should be treated with the appropriate antibiotics.

Thrombocytopenia – reduced platelet count. A count below 60000/mm^3 (60 × 10^9/litre) will lead to an increased risk of haemorrhage.

Purpura. Haemorrhage of the skin and mucous membranes.

Anaemia
Reduction in the number of circulating red blood cells, the haemoglobin level is often below 9g/dl.
May occur in malignant disease involving the bone marrow, in Hodgkin's Disease, hypersplenism and following prolonged haemorrhage.

Patients may complain of
Malaise

Lassitude
Headache
Amenorrhoea.
Patients will appear pale.

Nursing care includes
Adequate rest
Care of the skin, mouth and teeth
Attention to diet
Antianaemic drugs – as prescribed by Medical Officer

RADIATION EFFECTS ON THE GONADS AND FETUS

Radiation doses as low as 10 cGy can cause fetal abortion in early pregnancy.

In later pregnancy when organogenesis is taking place, malformations may be seen in the newborn infant.

If it is necessary to irradiate a pregnant female, the fetus should be protected from the radiation.

If the pregnancy is under 20 weeks, the possibility of an abortion may be considered. However, this is a subject which must be thought over very carefully by all who are involved medically with the patient and her husband and each case should be assessed individually.

Ovarian effects
In the early developing ovarian follicle, the oocyte and the granulosa cells are very radiosensitive.

Radiation effects on the ovaries depend on the dose received and the age of the female. The younger the woman, the greater the dose has to be to achieve a particular effect. Deliberate suppresion of ovarian function – a radiation induced menopause may be carried out for several reasons

To suppress ovarian hormones in malignant disease which has a hormone dependancy e.g. some breast cancers.

To suppress ovarian hormones associated with menstrual problems e.g. menorrhagia.

Indirect suppression may occur when irradiating the pelvis or abdomen for other malignant disease.

Care of the patient
Careful explanation of the effects to the patient and husband. Warned that suppression is not an immediate effect and con-

traception should be continued, if necessary, for up to 18 months.
Consent form should be signed by patient, before commencement
of treatment.
Patients may experience menopausal symptoms e.g. hot flushes,
vaginal dryness following radiotherapy.
Diarrhoea may be a problem, depending on the area of treatment
and the radiation dosage (see section on bowel reactions).

Testicular effects
Spermatogonia are very radiosensitive.
Permanent sterility will occur if the testis receives a dose of 500
cGy.
The interstitial cells which produce testosterone are not affected at
these dose levels.

Care of the patient
Patients should be told of the side effects of radiation to the testi-
cles.
Provision for the use of a sperm bank for these patients.

Genetic mutations
Very low doses, radiation levels too low to affect mitosis in the
gonads, can affect the genes, from which chromosomes are made,
leading to genetic mutations in any offspring. It is therefore important for student radiographers to understand how to prevent
the ovaries and testes from receiving radiation which could lead to
genetic mutation in later generations, therefore radiotherapy for
the treatment of non-malignant disease in the younger generation
is only used if other forms of treatment have proved unsuccessful.

RADIATION EFFECTS ON THE EYE

May be seen following radiotherapy to the eye:
    primary treatment for an orbital tumour or
    carcinoma of the antrum, involving the orbit
Retina is not radiosensitive at radiotherapy dosages.
Cornea, conjunctiva and the lens are more radiosensitive.
Eyelids are affected in the same way as the skin.

Conjunctiva
Conjunctival hyperaemia occurs soon after radiotherapy commences.

Swelling may lead to conjunctivitis, the columnar epithelium becomes keratinized.
Scarring may develop.

Care of the patient
To help prevent permanent damage, infection must be prevented with antibiotics e.g. gentamicin or chloramphenicol eye ointment

Lacrimal glands
Reduction or absence of secretions leads to 'dry eye' syndrome
May lead to keratitis, infection and ulceration

Care of the patient
Antibiotics prescribed to combat infection on the conjunctiva
Artificial tear solutions

Cornea
Corneal oedema and keratitis, worsened if lacrimal glands are affected.

Care of the patient
Keep inflammation to a minimum
Antibiotics prescribed

The ocular lens
X and gamma radiation doses of more than 200 cGy to the lens can cause cataract formation.
Radiation affects mitotic activity in the germinative zone of lens epithelium.
Epithelial cells differentiate into lens fibres, in the posterior capsule, swell up to form large, balloon like cells, developing into cataracts.
The damaged cells migrate to region of posterior pole and increase in size.
If the damaged area cannot be limited by repair processes, the opacity will involve the whole lens.

Care of the patient
The obvious treatment is prevention.
The dose to the lens is minimised by accurate beam direction and shielding of the lens with the appropriate thickness of lead.
Use may be made of the 'build-up' region on megavoltage which

may allow the maximum dose to be delivered posterior to the
lens.
If cataracts do appear, the only treatment is surgical resection.

RADIATION SICKNESS

A general reaction occuring during large field radiotherapy to
widespread or bulky tumours.
These tumours may affect the patient with their own metabolic
activities and by diversion of necessary nutrients to the tumour.
Following radiotherapy, these cellular, bulky tumours can produce excess nucleic acid, which need to be excreted by the kidneys.
The radiotherapy will also affect normal tissues.
All the factors together produce a clinical picture of radiation sick-
ness.

Care of the patient
Careful explanation should be given to the patient before treatment
commences

Tiredness	– ensure plenty of rest
Nausea or vomiting	– antiemetics – pyridoxine (Vitamin B6)
	stemetil (prochlorperazine)
	avomine (promethazine
	theoclate)
Anorexia	– small nourishing meals
	high fluid intake should be maintained
Headache/	
general aches and pains	– suitable analgesic

SUMMARY

The above section on radiation reactions is by no means complete.
It is intended to help the student radiographers realise the need
for a high standard of patient care if radiation side effects are to
be kept to a minimum. Not included in this section are the effects
of radiation on organs such as kidneys, lungs and the central nervous system, which are of no less importance. Radiographers need
to understand how to minimise all radiation effects on all normal
tissues, but this section is intended primarily to look at some of
the radiation effects which occur during the course of radiotherapy, which then come under the care of the radiographer.

Further reading on this complex subject can be obtained in the following books:

Coggle J E 1971 Biological Effects of Radiation, Wykeham Publications, London and Winchester
Duncan W, Nias A H W 1977 Clinical Radiogiology, Churchill Livingstone, Edinburgh
Lerman S 1980 Radiant Energy and the Eye, Balliere Tindall, New York
Walter J, Miller H, Bamford C K 1979 A Short Textbook of Radiotherapy, Churchill Livingstone, Edinburgh
Lowry S 1974 Fundamentals of Radiation Therapy, English Universities Press Limited, London

CARE OF THE PATIENT DURING SPECIAL PROCEDURES

KNIFE BIOPSY

Bios – life
Opsis – vision

A knife biopsy is carried out to obtain a section of skin/subcutaneous tissue for histological examination e.g. confirmation of diagnosis of a basal carcinoma of the skin, malignant skin deposits from a breast carcinoma.

If a small lesion is suspected of being a basal cell carcinoma the whole lesion can be completely excised either by a scalpel or a curette (Excision biopsy).

Duties of the radiographer
To prepare the biopsy trolley
To care for the patient before, during and after the procedure
To assist the radiotherapist during the procedure

Trolley setting
Wash hands thoroughly, dry on a paper towel
Shelves and rails sprayed with disinfectant
Dried with a sterile towel

Non sterile equipment
On the bottom shelf place
   Specimen jar
   Receiver for soiled dressing
   Antiseptic sprays
   Adhesive sprays
   Adhesive tape
Wash hands, dry

Sterile equipment

This should be set out as near to the time of the biopsy as possible to prevent contamination of the equipment by an airborne route. On the top shelf open a toilet and suture pack containing:

Outer coverings and dressing towels

Gallipots, two, which should contain an antiseptic e.g. Savlon (1/200) for skin sterilisation and one containing sterile water for rinsing any equipment such as the anaesthetic capsule which may have been sterilised in 1/30 Savlon

Gauze swabs and cotton wool balls.

Selection of forceps: Spencer Wells
                                   dissecting forceps

Scalpel or curette (previously sterilised)

Suture needle and silk

Scissors

Syringe, needle and local anaesthetic (lignocaine)

Surgeons gloves (disposable)

The top of the trolley is covered with a sterile towel.

Patient care

Reassure the nervous patient

Help the patient onto the couch

Remove any clothing as necessary from the patient

Explain the procedure to the patient

Reassure the patient throughout the procedure

Assist with the aftercare of the patient

Check that the dressing is secure

Arrange further appointments for follow up and for the removal of any stitches.

The radiographer should also

Check that the form accompanying the biopsy specimen has been completed by the radiotherapist and that it accompanies the specimen which is also correctly labelled

Tidy the room afterwards

THE PATHOLOGY FORM

A form requesting a pathological report on a specimen sent for examination.

For example

Specimen – blood,

Request– blood count

Specimen – skin and underlying tissue
Request– histology
The form should include the following details
  Hospital
  Department or Ward
  Medical officer in charge of the patient
  Nature of specimen
  Examination requested
  Clinical data of the patient
  Present treatment
Patient details
  Hospital number
  Surname
  Forenames
  Sex
  Age
  Ethnic origin
  Date and time specimen was taken
  Signature of the Medical Officer
Pathology
  Report number
  Date the specimen was received
  Time the specimen was received
  Full pathology report
Two copies
  One sent to Medical Officer
  One retained in Pathology Department

TROLLEY SETTING FOR A PELVIC EXAMINATION

This is a socially clean procedure (not sterile)
Trolley cleaned with antiseptic solution
Dried
Covered with a clean disposable towel

Articles placed on the trolley
Gloves
Lubricant (KY jelly)
Sponge holding forceps
Vulsellum forceps
Vaginal speculum
Proctoscope (if rectal examination is needed)
Gallipot with antiseptic solution

Swabs
Lamp
Receiver for soiled dressings and instruments
Spatula
Glass slides and cover slips
Sanitary towel

Duties of the radiographer
Prepare the trolley
Explain procedure to the patient
Assist patient with undressing and positioning
Reassure patient during the procedure
Act as chaperone for male medical staff
Arrange patient appointment and further transport
Tidy the room

TROLLEY SETTING FOR AN INDIRECT LARYNGOSCOPY

This is an indirect inspection of the larynx which is done during a course of radical radiotherapy to the larynx so that the radiation reaction can be assessed, and at follow up appointments to check on the results of the radiotherapy.
This is a clean procedure (not sterile)

Requirements
Large instrument tray with:
   Laryngeal mirror
   Spatula
   Paper towels and gauze swabs
   Finger stalls
Also required are
   Cocaine spray (to anaesthetise the throat)
   Spirit lamp and matches (to warm the laryngeal mirror)
   Bowl for dentures
   Mouth wash for patient
   Receiver for dirty swabs
   Head mirror – this is worn by the radiotherapist
      to reflect the light from behind the patient on to the laryngeal
      mirror in the throat.
If an infection is thought to be present the following are needed:
   Throat swab

Labels
Pathological request form

Duties of the radiographer
Prepare the trolley
Position the patient prior to the procedure
Assist the radiotherapist throughout the procedure
Reassure the patient throughout
Tidy the trolley afterwards
Lock away the benzocaine spray
Arrange transport if necessary
Arrange appointments if necessary
Check the forms if a throat swab has been taken

TROLLEY SETTING FOR AN INJECTION OF RADIOACTIVE PHOSPHORUS (^{32}P)

An intravenous injection of ^{32}P can be given as part of the treatment of polycythaemia rubra vera.
Sterile procedure therefore the trolley is prepared as described previously.
On the upper shelf place the following sterile equipment
  Dressing towel
  Gallipots containing – Savlon (1/200) for skin sterilisation
  Syringe of appropriate size for the injection
  Selection of swabs and cotton wool balls
Lower shelf
  Tourniquet
  Selection of disposable needles
  Surgeons gloves (disposable) – prior to opening
  Plastic apron
  Dressings for the injection site following the procedure
  Receiver for dirty (non-contaminated) dressings
  Plastic bag or special receiver for contaminated articles
  Specially coated protective sheeting with an absorbing side and a waterproof side e.g. 'Benchkote'
  Geiger counter

Duties of the radiographer
Prepare the trolley
Prepare the room – placing the absorbant sheeting in the appropriate places

Check that the correct amount of ^{32}P has been ordered and delivered

An intravenous dose of 150–220 megabecquerels (MBq) is usually the standard

Assist the patient into correct position

Assist the radiotherapist during the procedure

Release the tourniquet when the vein for injection has been located and the needle is in position

Reassure the patient throughout the procedure

After the procedure has finished

Tidy the room

Remove the contaminated articles to the appropriate protection area

Check that the patients' wound has stopped bleeding

Check the room and staff for contamination using the geiger counter

Check patient for contamination (other than at the injection site)

Arrange for transport

Arrange a follow up appointment

Store unused ^{32}P in the protected area.

TRAY AND TROLLEY SETTING FOR INJECTION OF RADIOACTIVITY YTTRIUM 90(^{90}Y) INTO THE PLEURAL CAVITY

The presence of tumour deposits in the pleural cavity stimulates the pleura to produce excess fluid. This results in the patient experiencing breathing difficulty which is extremely distressing. The excess fluid must first be removed and then the tumour can be treated. One method of treatment is to inject into the pleural cavity, a radioactive fluid such as Yttrium 90, which will irradiate the tumour deposits with beta rays of energy 2·26 megavolts (MeV).

Dosage calculations are complex but 1,110MBq of ^{90}Y delivers a uniform tumour lethal dose to the pleural cavity.

Trolley setting

Sterile procedure therefore the trolley is prepared as described previously.

On top shelf place the following

　　Large syringe (50 cc)

　　Selection of steel needles

Two way tap
Rubber tubing (to fit the tap)
Collecting receiver with Savlon (to collect excess pleural fluid)
Gallipot and antiseptic solution
Swabs
Forceps, artery forceps to clamp on to needle when injecting radioactive fluid, this prevents the needle from being pushed further into the cavity
Selection of sterile towels
Local anaesthetic e.g. Lignocaine 0·5%
Needle and syringe

Other articles include
Surgeons disposable gloves
Face mask
Plastic apron for staff protection
Plastic bag for receiving contaminated waste
Bag for receiving dirty swabs
Facilities should be available for colouring the colourless radioactive solution (by Physicist)
A sterile saline solution may be injected afterwards to make sure that all the radioactive solution has been injected

Duties of the radiographer
Prepare the trolley
Arrange for the preparation of the radioactive solution
Explain the procedure to the patient
Assist the patient with undressing and positioning
Patient usually put in sitting position
Arms resting on some support (couch)
Procedure carried out from the back of the patient which allows access to the costo diaphragmatic recess
Reassure the patient throughout the procedure
Assist radiotherapist during procedure

After the procedure has finished
Assist patient, the procedure can take a long time and can be tiring
Clean the trolley
Remove contaminated articles to the appropriate protection area
Check the room and staff for contamination
Check the patient for contamination (other than injection area)
Return the patient to the ward

TRAY AND TROLLEY SETTING FOR INJECTION OF RADIOACTIVE YTTRIUM 90 (^{90}Y) INTO ABDOMINAL CAVITY

Tumour deposits create the same problems as in the pleural cavity. The treatment policy is therefore the same.

Extremely large amounts of fluid can be tolerated in the peritoneal cavity without too much discomfort, therefore drainage can take up to an hour.

Trolley setting

Sterile procedure and therefore the trolley is prepared as described previously.

On top shelf place the following
Seldinger trocar and cannula
Two way tap
Forceps, tissue
Spencer Wells artery forceps
Scalpel – incision is made prior to introduction of trocar and cannula
Suture needle and silk – for sewing up the wound afterwards
Swabs
Gallipot containing antiseptic solution
Scissors
Syringe, needle and local anaesthetic solution
Rubber tubing and funnel (fluid is not injected with a syringe but run in slowly through a funnel)
Selection of sterile towels

Other articles include
Surgeons disposable gloves
Face mask
Plastic apron for staff protection
Plastic bag for receiving contaminated material
Bag for receiving dirty swabs etc.
Dye to colour the fluid
A small quantity of sterile saline solution may be used to flush the remaining radioactive solution through the funnel and tubing.

The duties of the radiographer

See previous section – page 79

Contamination checks the same, but the activity of the solution is often 2900–3700 MBq.

ALTERNATIVE TREATMENT METHODS

Because of the radiation hazards involved in the above procedures it is becoming more common to inject chemotherapy drugs into the cavity, following drainage procedures.

Examples

Pleural effusion
Excess fluid removed from the pleural cavity by slow suction pump (over 48 hours)
Bleomycin 60–120 mg, in 100 ml saline is then injected into the cavity
After 24 hours the fluid is evacuated

Peritoneal effusion
Excess fluid from the peritoneal cavity is gravity drained over 6–24 hours
Bleomycin 60–120 mg, in 100 ml normal saline is then instilled into the cavity.

CARE OF THE PATIENT UNDERGOING CHEMOTHERAPY

INTRODUCTION

The use of cytotoxic drugs now plays a major role in the treatment of malignant disease. Radiographers have in their care, patients undergoing chemotherapy and radiotherapy and therefore need to understand the side effects of both of these treatments if the patient is to receive the best care and attention.

To discuss all cytotoxic drugs and their side effects would be impossible and probably soon out of date therefore, the aim is to discuss the common side effects of cytotoxic therapy.

Each drug has individual toxic actions but one property is common to all of them and that is they are unable to distinguish between normal and malignant cells. This means that when a cytotoxic drug is in the body it will attack all cells and so it is necessary to minimise the damage to the normal cells whilst enhancing the toxic effect on the malignant cells

GROUPS OF CYTOTOXIC AGENTS

Alkylating agents

Mode of action within the cell
The drugs replace the hydrogen bond between the DNA bases with a hydrocarbon (alkylation). It is thought that this action prevents these base areas from acting as templates for new DNA replication.

Alkylation of enzymes in the cell prevents them from fulfilling their role in DNA replication.

Examples
Nitrogen mustard
Cyclophosphamide
Melphalan
Chlorambucil

Antimetabolites

Mode of action within the cell
Metabolites are incorporated into new proteins and nucleic acid prior to mitosis.

Antimetabolite cytotoxic drugs chemically resemble these metabolites and are taken into the nucleus. The cell is then incapable of protein synthesis, or forms protein not able to function as required by the cell.

Examples
Methotrexate   – prevents purine and pyrimidine synthesis
5 Fluorouracil   – prevents pyrimidine synthesis
Cytosine arabinoside – prevents pyrimidine synthesis
6 Mercaptopurine   – prevents purine synthesis
N.B. Purines and pyrimidines are essential constituents of DNA and RNA.

Compounds of biological origin

Mode of action within the cell
Not clear.

Thought to act in the early stage of cell division by interfering with RNA and DNA synthesis.

Examples
Vincristine
Vinblastine

Antimitotic antibiotics

Mode of action within the cell
Attaches itself to a DNA molecule at the site where transfer RNA usually functions, preventing the DNA from reduplicating.

All the antibiotic cytotoxic drugs potentiate the action of radiotherapy leading to extreme skin reactions when both are used.

Examples
Actinomycin D
Mitomycin C
Adriamycin
Bleomycin

Miscellaneous

Asparaginase. Destroys all free asparagine in the body.

Asparagine is an amino acid essential to all cells. Malignant cells cannot make asparagine, therefore this drug exploits a biochemical difference between normal and malignant cells.

Value has proved limited because of severe toxicity and a rapid resistance to the drug.

Nitrosoureas – BCNU (bis-chloroethyl nitrosourea) and CCNU (Chloroethyl-cyclohexyl nitrosourea).

Often classed as alkylating agents, but they also inhibit mitosis by blocking certain enzymes necessary for purine synthesis.

GENERAL PRINCIPLES

Cytotoxic drugs may be used as:

A curative treatment
e.g. Chorioncarcinoma, a malignant tumour of the placenta, can be successfully treated in the early stages with methotrexate and actinomycin D.

An adjuvant to surgery/radiotherapy
e.g. Nephroblastoma of the kidney is now treated using a combination of surgery, radiotherapy and cytotoxic therapy – actinomycin D, which has dramatically increased the survival rate.

A palliative treatment when other treatment methods have failed
e.g. Metastatic carcinoma of the breast when surgery, radiotherapy and hormone therapy have failed to control the disease.

GENERALISED SIDE EFFECTS FROM THE USE OF CYTOTOXIC THERAPY

Bone marrow depression

Some drugs cause an immediate drop in the blood count by affecting the cells already in the blood (limited effect).

Other drugs affect the stem cells in the bone marrow leading to delayed effects in the peripheral blood.

Leucopenia occurs first.

Life span of leucocytes averages 5 days, therefore the effects are seen in under a week.

Care of the patient

There is increased risk of contracting infection

Treatment is suspended if white cell count falls to $2 \cdot 0 \times 10^9$/litre

Bone marrow is allowed to recover

Patients warned about the risk of infection

If white blood count drops very low following intensive treatment, the patient may have to be reverse barrier nursed.

Pyrexia could indicate that infection is present

A broad spectrum antibiotic can be given until the infection has been identified.

Thrombocytopenia

A reduction of circulating blood platelets

Can be seen two weeks after the start of chemotherapy

Care of the patient

Treatment is suspended if the platelet count falls to 50×10^9/litre

Patients warned of the risk of haemorrhage therefore electric razors should be used

Problems with menstruation
Sudden epistaxis   } inform the medical officer
General body bruising

Erythrocytopenia

Not normally seen after cytotoxic therapy

Red blood cells have a life span of 120 days

Effects would not be seen for several months – meanwhile the bone marrow should be recovering from the treatment

If the haemoglobin level is below 9 g/dl, a blood transfusion is given.

Epilation

Many drugs are capable of causing hair loss

Vincristine and adriamycin are particularly toxic to the hair follicles

Has the same psychological effect as with radiation induced hair loss

Scalp hair is more sensitive to damage than other body hair

Regrowth readily occurs as the follicles quickly develop a resistance to the drugs

It is necessary to provide wigs during the epilation period.

Gastrointestinal effects

Effects depend on the drugs used and the dose

Bleomycin and methotrexate cause soreness of the mucosal lining of the mouth and pharynx leading to painful ulceration.

Care of the patient

Glycerin and thymol mouthwashes

Careful use of toothbrushes

Benzocaine emulsion given before meals

Attention to diet – soft, bland food

High fluid intake

For infections – antibiotic therapy e.g. tetracycline syrup

If thrush develops – nystatin emulsion

Dental caries may be precipitated by cytotoxic therapy

Carious teeth should be removed beforehand

Nausea and vomiting are often a problem

Some drugs irritate the gastric lining e.g. BCNU (bis-chloroethyl nitrosourea)

Some stimulate the vomiting centre in the brain e.g. nitrogen mustard

Patients have been known to vomit at the thought of having cytotoxic therapy

Antiemetics should be prescribed

A light diet should be advised

Diarrhoea is controlled with the appropriate drugs e.g. imodium capsules

A high fluid intake is recommended.

Reproductive system

Many cytotoxic drugs suppress spermatogenesis and oogenesis

Alkylating agents are particularly toxic

Provision of sperm banks for the male patients
Female patients should be warned of irregular menstrual cycle.

Genetic mutations

The effect of cytotoxic therapy on the chromosomes is not fully understood
Effects may become more apparent with increasing use of cytotoxic therapy and an increase in the number of long term survivors
During pregnancy it is thought unwise to give treatment during the first three months and methotrexate and the alkylating agents are absolutely contraindicated during this period.

Hyperuricaemia

Excess uric acid in the blood stream
Caused by breakdown of purine bases of DNA
Uric acid cannot be destroyed in the body, therefore it must be excreted
Toxic effects of excess uric acid includes renal damage and swollen joints (gout)
Occurs where there has been rapid breakdown of a large number of tumour cells due to chemotherapy or radiotherapy
Treatment – allopurinol converts the uric acid into a less toxic form for excretion.

Immunosuppression

Majority of cytotoxic drugs are known to suppress the body's immune response system
Patients are more susceptible to infections and can cope less readily with any invading pathogen
It is thought that a long term effect is the risk of developing a new malignancy because of the immunosuppression
This may prove to be important as more patients are treated and surviving for many years.

11

Drugs

INTRODUCTION

Patients attending an X-ray or radiotherapy department may be receiving a variety of drugs. Although drug prescribing is the province of the medical staff, radiographers should have enough knowledge to understand the effects of drugs and what may happen if the patient has forgotten to take a particular drug or has taken too much in error.

This section is intended as a brief outline of the complex data of drug classification and examples of each category. Drugs used in the departments should be familiar to all staff and their desired effects and side effects understood. Student radiographers should know the principles behind the use of addictive drugs and the importance of following the strict procedures for the ordering, storage and administration of these drugs.

It is anticipated that students will obtain the widest experience of the use of drugs during their ward experience.

Drugs are substances used for medicinal purposes, they can be a source of danger to the patient if taken in sufficient quantity.

LAWS CONTROLLING DRUGS

Medicines Act (111) 1968

This act states that all medicines, except those on the General Sale List, may only be sold or supplied from registered pharmacies. The drugs covered under this act are classified as follows:

General Sale List medicines (G.S.L.)

This section applies to retail pharmacies. Drugs on this list can be sold in such places as supermarkets, but only in specific conditions e.g. drugs should be prepacked and not sold loose.

Examples of drugs covered – Aspro, dental cream.

Pharmacy medicines (P)

This section applies to retail pharmacies. Drugs on this list are under partial control and may only be sold if a pharmacist is present. The pharmacist can then advise when and how to use the drugs, and, if necessary, on any side effects which may occur.

Examples of drugs covered – Dulcolax suppositories, insulin.

Prescription only Medicines (P.O.M.)

Drugs on this list must have a written prescription, signed in indelible ink, by a Doctor or Dentist.

Examples of drugs covered – Adrenalin, Gastrografin.

Misuse of Drugs Act 1971

Drugs mentioned by this Act used to be called Dangerous Drugs and are now called Controlled Drugs (CD) and are in four categories.

Marked CD Intravenous (Schedule 1)

These drugs have negligible risk of abuse, therefore there is no restriction on administration.

Examples of drugs covered – Codeine and morphine combined with other substances.

Marked CD (Schedule 2)

These drugs can only be administered by a Doctor, Dentist or nurse.
Examples of drugs covered – Opiates e.g. heroin, morphine
Major stimulants e.g. amphetamines

Marked CD No Register (Schedule 3)

These drugs are not so harmful as drugs in Schedules 2 and 4.

Examples of drugs covered – Minor stimulants e.g. benzphetamine.

Marked CD Licence (Schedule 4)

These drugs have virtually no therapeutic value and are not held in hospitals.

Examples of drugs covered – Hallucinogenic drugs e.g. Cannabis, L.S.D.

CONTAINERS AND LABELS

Containers

Can be

Coloured bottles with child-proof lids

Ampoules

Bottles with rubber tops, the contents are removed with a syringe and needle, after the top has been cleaned with a sterile solution

Ridged bottles – always contain poisons which are not for internal use

Labels

Must be

Indelible

In English

Must state

Name of the preparation

Name of the patient

Directions for use

Name and address of the supplier

Keep out of reach of children

UNITS OF MEASUREMENT

Milligrams	– mg
Grams	– g
Millilitres	– ml
Litres	– l
Weight/volume	– % strength

ADMINISTRATION

All drugs should be checked against the name of the patient.

When the drug is removed from the cupboard

When measuring the dose of the drug

Before giving the drug to the patient

By mouth

For each patient check the prescription, drug, dose and strength.

Medicine

Shake the bottle (unless stated otherwise)

Remove the stopper or screw cap

Hold with the label uppermost

Pour into the glass at eye level

Ensure the patient takes the drug

Tablets

Check the number of tablets

Place the tablets in a container – no touch technique
Ensure the patient takes the tablets
In both cases record that the drug has been taken

Disadvantages of the oral method
The patient may refuse to swallow the drug
The drug is only partially absorbed
The drug may irritate the stomach causing vomiting/diarrhoea

Per rectum
For each patient check the prescription, drug, dose and strength.
The drug may be in the form of
   Suppositories e.g. Dulcolax
   Enemas   e.g. Barium sulphate
   Anaesthetic   e.g. Sodium thiopentone

Inhalation
For each patient check the prescription, drug, dose and strength.
The drug may be in the form of either a vapour, liquid, gas, often
used for respiratory tract infections.
   For example antispasmodic drugs for asthma e.g. Bextasol
                  anaesthetic gases e.g. nitrous oxide

Injection
For each patient check the prescription, drug, dose and strength.

Trolley setting
Disposable cannula
          syringe
          needle
Drug
Skin cleanser e.g. Mediswabs
Adhesive dressing
Bag for dirty swabs
'Sharps box' for needles and empty ampoules
Emergency drugs
also arm support
Tourniquet may be required

Intravenous injection
The drug may only be administered by a doctor if this route is
used

Reasons for the route
    Quick acting in an emergency
    Drug introduced into the circulatory system e.g. for diagnostic purposes
    Anaesthetics may be introduced
Sites
    Midcubital vein of the forearm
    Scalp veins
Container – Ampoules
Method
    Explain the procedure to the patient
    Reassure the patient
    Show the doctor the ampoule prior to opening it
    Apply the tourniquet
    Support the arm
    Clean the skin
    Ask the patient to open and close their hand – to distend the veins in the elbow region
    Doctor inserts the sterile needle
    Release the tourniquet prior to the injection
After the injection
    Apply swab and digital pressure to the puncture site
    Apply an adhesive dressing
    Dispose of the needle and ampoule in the sharps box
    Dispose of the syringe and swabs
    Put away the rest of the equipment

Infusion
Allows the administration of large quantities of fluid, via a 'giving set' (Fig. 11.1) which controls the rate of flow, the solution may be given over a period of between 30 minutes and several days depending on the drug used.
Site   – Midcubital vein of the forearm
Containers – Bottle, bag
Method   – See intravenous injection

Care of the infusion set
    Ensure
    No contamination of the apparatus
    No air bubbles in the tubing
    Infusion bag is clamped correctly
    Drip is running through correctly

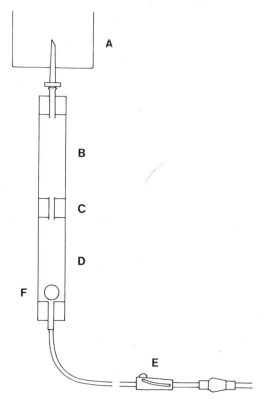

Fig. 11.1   Drip infusion set
A – Drug in solution in a plastic container
B – Filter chamber
C – Drip chamber
D – Float chamber
E – Flow control
F – Float-ball

The bag is kept at the correct height above the patient
There is no patient reaction to the drug
Avoid
Straining the infusion set
Trapping the tubing
Dislodging the needle
Reconnecting a broken system
Examples
Chemotherapy drugs
Contrast agent e.g. Biligram infusion
Electrolyte solutions

Subcutaneous injection

This route is used when a small quantity of fluid is introduced 'under the skin'.

Sites   – Outer aspect of the upper arm, thigh

Container – Usually has a rubber top so that small quantities may be withdrawn

Method

Explain the procedure to the patient

Reassure the patient

Wipe the bottle top with alcohol swab

Check and withdraw the required quantity of the drug

Change the needle

Swab the skin

Administer and record that the injection has been given

Examples – Adrenalin, Insulin

Intramuscular injection

This route is used when large quantities of fluid are introduced.

Sites

Outer aspect of the shoulder

Antero-lateral aspect of the upper thigh

Upper, outer aspect of the buttocks

Container

Ampoules

Method

Explain the procedure to the patient

Reassure the patient

Check and open the ampoule, using a sterile swab to hold the top

Using a cannula, withdraw the drug

Replace the cannula with a needle

Swab the skin

Administer and record.

Examples

Penicillin, Morphine, Atropine

CONTROLLED DRUGS (CD and CD Licenced)

These must be kept in a locked cupboard, inside another locked cupboard, a red light may indicate when the door is open. State Registered nurses hold the keys, each nurse holding the key for 1 cupboard. Two people must witness that the drug has been administered, one of whom must be a doctor or a State Registered nurse.

Procedure

Collect the written prescription and the record book

Check that the patient has not already taken the prescribed dose of the drug

Select the drug and check the contents with the total in the book

Check the dose and the drug remaining in the container

Relock the drugs cupboard

Enter patients name, dose of drug and the date given in the record book

Take the prescription and the drugs to the patient and recheck the quantity and the drug

Adminster the drug to the patient

Enter the exact time of administration in the book

Both witnesses sign the book.

DRUGS FOR PATIENT PREPARATION FOR DIAGNOSTIC EXAMINATIONS

Aperients and suppositories – used for bowel preparation

Sedatives – used to calm the patient

Premedications – used to relax the patient and reduce secretions prior to a general anaesthetic, may reduce postoperative vomiting

Local anaesthetic – used to stop sensation in a localised area

Analgesics – used to reduce pain

Contrast agents – used to outline organs in radiography

RESUSCITATION DRUGS .

Adrenalin – for injection, raises the blood pressure

Analaptic drugs – to stimulate and restore e.g.

Aminophylline – stimulates respiration

Methedrine – stimulates central nervous system

Nikethamide – stimulates the heart and respiration

Antihistamines – reduce allergic reaction e.g.

Piriton

Phenergan

Anthisan

ANAESTHETIC GASES

Nitrous oxide – cylinder is blue (anaesthetic)

Carbon dioxide – cylinder is grey (repiratory stimulant)

Entox (oxygen and nitrous oxide) – cylinder is blue with a white and blue top (anaesthetic)
Oxygen – cylinder is black with a white cuff

CONTRAST AGENTS

Air
Carbon dioxide
Barium sulphate
Iodine based compounds

12

Radiographic contrast agents

INTRODUCTION

During the course of their work, student radiographers will come into contact with many types of contrast agents, but because of individual radiological preferences, and the number of agents available, students may find that other agents or dosages are used in the departments in which they work. For the safety of the patient and the success of the examination, it is important that students understand the contraindications for the various contrast agents and to know why the specific agents are used.

Contrast agents are substances which can be used to demonstrate organs, vessels and parts of the body more clearly.

PRINCIPLES OF ACTION OF RADIOGRAPHIC CONTRAST AGENTS

As the atomic weights (total weight of protons and neutrons) of substances vary, the rate of absorption of X-radiation also varies.

The denser the substance the more the radiation is attenuated. Contrast agents may be of 2 types:

Negative – Have a low atomic weight and therefore provide a negative contrast on the film as they absorb very little radiation.

Positive – Have a high atomic weight and therefore provide a positive contrast on the film as they absorb most of the radiation.

NEGATIVE CONTRAST AGENTS

Air

This may be introduced by the patient e.g.

Chest radiographs – taken on inspiration, air in the lungs gives good tissue detail.

Valsalva manoeuvre – forced expiration on a closed glottis (alternative, asking the patient to breath out, holding the air in the cheeks). Outlines the trachea.

Air or oxygen

Both gases can be retained by the body for a long period of time

Used if tomography is required

There is a danger of gas embolism forming

Air is introduced through a sterile swab to filter it.

e.g. Air encephalography 30–40 mls of air or oxygen.

   Arthrography 30–40 mls of air or oxygen.

If gas embolism occurs

   Patient is placed on their left side

   The head is lowered

   Oxygen is given under positive pressure

   Cardiac arrest may occur, if so, cardiac massage is performed

   Patient must not sit up for several hours

Carbon dioxide

Less risk of gas embolism

Rapidly absorbed (within 45 minutes)

e.g. *Barium meals* – to provide a double contrast with the barium, can be in tablet, liquid, powder, or the carbon dioxide is ready mixed with the barium sulphate.

POSITIVE CONTRAST AGENTS

Barium sulphate

Introduced orally, per rectum, or as a sterile solution to demonstrate the urinary bladder.

Table 12.2   Example of the use of barium sulphate

Examination	Consistency
Barium swallow	
for cardiac outline	Barium paste
for oesophagus	Barium sulphate (100% W/V)
Barium meal	Barium sulphate (250% W/V)
Small bowel enema	Barium sulphate and water
Barium enema	Barium sulphate (60% W/V)
Cystography	Sterile barium sulphate

Contraindications

Suspected fistula or sinus – because the barium sulphate is not absorbed by the body

Sometimes contraindicated prior to surgery – because the barium sulphate is not absorbed by the body

Additives
Flavouring – makes the agent more palatable for children

Drugs
Hyoscine-N-Butylbromide (Buscopan) – 20mg given intravenously enables the stomach/colon to be examined free of muscle spasm
Metoclopromide (Maxolon) – 10mg given intravenously to co-ordinate peristaltic movement and therefore aids gastric emptying.

Iodine compounds

Methods of introduction
Ingestion
Intravenous injection
Drip infusion
Catheterisation

Table 12.3 Classification Organic iodine compounds.

Examination	Active agent	Trade example	Example dosage
Angiography	Meglumine iothalamate	Conray 420	20 – 50 ml
	Sodium diatrizoate and		
	meglumine diatrizoate	Urografin 370	30 – 50 ml
Urography	Metrizoate salts	Triosil	50 ml
	Sodium diatrizoate	Hypaque 25	50 ml
		Hypaque 45	50 ml
	Meglumine diatrizoate and		
	Sodium diatrizoate	Urografin 290	50 ml
Biliary tract			
Infusion	Meglumine ioglycamide	Biligram	100 ml
Oral	Iopanoic acid	Telepaque	3 g
		Cistobil	3 g
Alimentary tract	Sodium diatrizoate and	Gastrografin	60 – 80 ml
	meglumine diatrizoate		
Radiculography	Metrizamide	Amipaque	10 ml
Myelography	Ethyl iodo-phenyl		
	undecyclate	Myodil	6 ml
Venography	Meglumine iothalamate	Conray 280	20 – 30 ml
	Meglumine diatrizoate	Urografin 310M	20 – 30 ml

Contraindications
Patient may have an allergy to iodine

Precautions

Check if the patient has any history of allergy/asthma/hay fever/
bronchitis
Have full resuscitation facilities available

Dosage

Varies according to:
   Patient's age
             condition
             weight
   Method of introduction
   Examination being undertaken
   Molecular size of the medium
   Children – dose according to body weight e.g. $1.0-1.2$ml/kg
   (maximum 25ml)

Administration

Record	– Dosage and any reaction
Doctor	– Checks name and concentration
	Introduces contrast agent
Observe	– For signs of reaction

Table 12.4   Iodized oils

Examination	Active agent	Trade example	Example dosage
Bronchography	Propyliodone and caroxymethyl cellulose	Dionosil aqueous	14 ml/lung
Lymphography	Iodised ethyl ester of fatty acids of poppy seed oil	Lipiodol ultra fluid	5 – 10 ml
Sialography	Iodised ethyl esters of fatty acids of poppy seed oil	Lipiodol	0.5 – 2 ml

13

First aid

INTRODUCTION

Patients attending an X-ray or radiotherapy department will experience a certain degree of stress which will add to their specific medical problem.

Together these problems may occasionally precipitate a medical emergency varying from dizziness and fainting to a cardiac arrest.

Radiographers who are looking after the patients must be able to recognise the signs and symptoms of medical emergencies and initiate the appropriate first aid action.

The ability to recognise a medical emergency and arrange for prompt treatment may well save a patient's life.

GENERAL PRINCIPLES OF FIRST AID

To sustain life
To prevent the condition from becoming worse
To promote patient recovery

ACTION SEQUENCE

If possible send for assistance (but do not leave the patient alone).
Check to see if the patient
   is breathing
   has a heart beat
   is bleeding
   has any broken bones
   has any burns
In all instances
   Send for medical aid as soon as possible
   Administer the appropriate first aid
      e.g. resuscitate
         arrest haemorrhage etc.
         (See later for specific details)

After care of the patient
Observe their – colour

> pulse
> respiratory rate
> level of consciousness

Always check for delayed shock.

After the emergency
Fill in an accident form
Report the incident to the superintendent in charge of the department
Report to the ward sister if the patient is an in patient
Report to the clinic if the patient is an out patient.

ACCIDENT FORMS

These should be completed as soon as possible after the accident and contain the following informmation:
  Name of hospital/department
  Name of the victim
  If member of staff/patient/visitor
  Home address
  Date of birth
If an employee has an accident
  Occupation
  Length of time absent from work (if any)
Details of the accident
  Nature and extent of injuries
  How the injuries were caused
  Where and when the accident occurred
If seen by a Doctor
  Note treatment prescribed and carried out
Witnesses their:
  Name
  Address
Equipment
  Description of equipment involved
  Action taken with regard to repair
Signatures of the
  Victim
  Member of staff in charge of the patient
Copies to the
  Victim
  Head of department
  Sector administrator.
  Occupational Health Department

FIRST AID TREATMENT

Condition	Cause	Signs and symptoms	First aid treatment
Shock occurs when the cardio-vascular system is incapabale of delivering oxygen and nutrients to the cells		Skin grey, cold, clammy Body temperature drops Muscles relax Pulse rate increases and is weak Respiration becomes rapid, shallow and sighing Nausea Lowered blood pressure Loss of consciousness	Establish and remove cause Reassure the patient Keep warm and comfortable Lie patient flat and raise the legs (unless contraindicated e.g. injured) Move gently Check airway (dentures) If vomiting place in the coma position.
Cardiogenic shock When the action of the heart is impaired	Disease of heart muscles Cardiac injury Heart failure		
Hypovolemic shock Loss of circulating blood volume	Haemorrhage Vomiting Diarrhoea Severe burns		
Neurogenic shock Loss of vascular tone and therefore dilatation of blood vessels	Severe pain Fright		Reassure the patient Keep them warm and comfortable.

Electric shock	High Voltage (up to 400kV)	May include:
		Cardiac arrest
		Respiratory failure
		Burns
		Fractures
		Shock
			DO NOT TOUCH EVEN IN-DIRECTLY UNLESS THE PA-TIENT HAS BEEN THROWN AWAY FROM THE SOURCE
			When isolated:
			Check airway–resuscitate if required
			Check pulse–resuscitate if required
			Treat: Bleeding
			        Fractures
			        Shock
			Report cause

	Low voltage
	(Domestic supply under 415V)
		see High voltage	Switch off current or break contact using an insulator e.g. a lead rubber apron.
			Check airway – resuscitate if required
			Check pulse – resuscitate if required
			Treat: Bleeding
			        Fractures
			        Shock
			Report cause
			Equipment safety check

Asphyxia A condition when no oxygen can be delivered to the body cells, therefore increase carbon dioxide tension	Obstruction Paralysis of the respiratory muscles Breathing a medium with no air e.g. Carbon monoxide	Breathing rate increased Cyanosis Noisy breathing, dyspnoea Loss of consciousness	Remove patient from the cause Clear airway Check airway – resuscitate if required Place in coma position

Condition	Cause	Signs and symptoms	First aid treatment
Burns	Dry heat e.g. fire electricity friction strong acids/alkalis	May include: Reddening of the skin Pain Blistering Destruction of skin and underlying tissue	Cover with dry, sterile dressing to reduce the risk of infection Treat for shock
Scalds	Moist heat	see Burns	see Burns Immerse in cold water if possible Remove clothing from body to prevent further scalding
Fainting	Temporarily inadequate supply of blood to the brain	Skin pale and clammy Perspiration on forehead Dizziness Ringing in ears Tingling in fingers Unconsciousness	Check airway Undo tight clothing Open windows Place head lower than feet Rub face and hands Give the patient a drink unless contraindicated
Convulsions Uncontrolled generalised movements which may be associated with loss of consciousness	Unknown	Twitching of limbs Cyanosis Stiffness Head and spine arched Breath held prior to the attack	Check airway Loosen tight clothing Fresh air
Epilepsy Type of convulsion	Brain tumour Metabolic disturbances		

Condition	Signs/Symptoms	Treatment
Petit Mal	Unconsciousness (short time) Pale Glassy expression in eyes Patient unaware of its occurence	None usually required
Grand Mal	Patient may have an aura *Tonic phase* Unconsciousness Muscle spasm Cyanosis Hands & teeth clenched Respiration ceases *Clonic phase* Contraction/relaxation Saliva may 'froth' from the lips $\frac{1}{2}$ – 2 minutes later relaxes Coma Patient wakens exhausted Sleeps Recovers consciousness May vomit	Clear space round patient Loosen clothing Remove spectacles Prevent patient from injuring themselves. When recovered allow to rest Do not send home unaccompanied
Jacksonian Epilepsy (focal epilepsy)	Brain tumour Encephalitis Following head injury	Patients starts twitching (toes and fingers first) Twitching continues over one side of body May/may not lose consciousness.	None usually required Usual care for unconscious patients
Foreign bodies	In the eye	Excessive watering	Cover with clean cloth Do not attempt to remove
	In the ear	? pain	Small quantities of oil may be poured in the ear

Condition	Cause	Signs and symptoms	First aid treatment
	In the nose	Snuffling	Cover with a clean, dry dressing To arrest bleeding apply indirect pressure
Poisoning	Corrosive substance e.g. phenol	Burns on lips and mouth Pain Vomiting Shock Thirst	Water or milk to drink
	Instant e.g. mercury arsenic	Pain in abdomen Vomiting blood Diarrhoea Collapse	Emetic – if cause is certain Gastric lavage If collapsed, warm abdomen
	Hypnotic and Neurotic e.g. morphine barbiturates	Drowsiness Coma Slow respirations	Give emetic Gastric lavage Artificial respiration Doctor required to give drugs to counteract e.g. methedrine
	Convulsant e.g. strychnine	Restlessness Delirium Convulsions	Give emetic Gastric lavage Rest Doctor required to give drugs to counteract e.g. scolene
	Carbon monoxide	See Asphyxia	See Asphyxia

14

Resuscitation procedure

INTRODUCTION

Following a cardiac arrest, irreversible brain damage will occur if the brain is starved of oxygen for more than three minutes. Successful application of external cardiac massage and artificial respiration must have saved countless numbers of lives.

It is unacceptable for a patient to die or be permanently mentally retarded after a cardiac arrest because of a lack of knowledge on resuscitation procedures by radiographers.

This section outlines the resuscitation procedure which should be known by every member of staff and every student. It would be of great value if the students are able to receive practical instruction on a special resuscitation dummy.

Special cardiac arrest teams, in hospitals, can be summoned by telephone, their telephone number should be known by everyone.

In all instances
  Never leave the patient
  Send for help
  Check pulse e.g. carotid pulse
  Check respiratory rate

CARDIAC ARREST

This is the failure of the heart to maintain the blood circulation.

Dangers
Brain damage occurs if circulatory supply is not restored within 3 minutes.

Signs and symptoms of cardiac arrest
Sudden collapse of the patient
No pulse (carotid or femoral)
Loss of consciousness

Cyanosis
Dilating or dilated pupils.

Procedure
Send for the cardiac arrest team
Precardiac percussion – sharp blow to lower end of sternum
Check pulse as the blow may have started the heart

If there is no pulse start cardiac massage
Clear airway
Hold chin forward – prevents displacement of the tongue
Ensure patient is on a hard surface
e.g. X-ray table/treatment couch/floor
Place heel of one hand over lower third of sternum in the midline
Place the other hand over first – see Fig. 14.1
Press HARD – sternum depressed 3–5 cm in an adult
Continue at a rate of 60/minute.

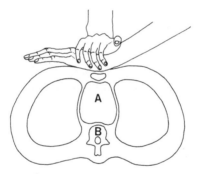

Fig. 14.1   Hand Position for Cardiac Massage
A – Heart
B – Thoracic vertebra

EXPIRED AIR RESUSCITATION – MOUTH TO MOUTH METHOD

This should be performed in conjunction with cardiac massage
e.g. 6 compressions to 1 ventilation.
   Check patient's airway
   Extend neck – head well back
   Pinch nose with one hand
   Support chin with the other hand
   Take a deep breath in
   Place mouth over patient's mouth forming a seal

Exhale – turn to watch chest inflate (if chest does not inflate – there could be an obstruction)
Continue at a rate of 12/minute.

If Brook airway available
Check that the airway is clear
Insert airway into the patient's mouth over the tongue into the back of the patient's mouth
Pinch patient's nose
Expand the patient's lungs via the airway (one way valve ensures patient's exhaled air escapes via the exit port).

If oxygen is available
Insert oral airway into the patient's mouth
Inlet of 'Ambu-bag' attached to the oxygen supply 10–15 litres/minute oxygen required
Patient's chin held foreward
Mask over patient's mouth forming a seal
Bag squeezed at the rate of 12/minute.

After the arrival of the cardiac arrest team, the following actions may be initiated

Defibrillation
Electrodes of defibrillator covered with jelly
1 placed over the patient's sternum
1 placed over the apex of the patient's heart
Ensure nobody is touching the table/patient
D.C. shock of 100 joules given (may be increased up to 400 joules)

Cardiac monitor
Patient attached to the monitor
Patient's cardiac rhythm can be observed

Table 14.1   Examples of drugs which may be given in cases of cardiac arrest

Diagnosis	Drug
Acidosis due to lack of respiration	Infusion – 100ml 8·4% Sodium bicarbonate
Sinus bradycardia	Intravenous Atropine 0·6 mg
Heart block	Intravenous Lignocaine 200 mg
	Practolol 10 mg
	Procainamide 200 mg
Asystole	Intravenous
	Adrenalin 1 ml of 1:1000
	Calcium gluconate 10 ml of 10%

15

Administration of oxygen

INTRODUCTION

Oxygen, either in cylinders or piped from the wall, is present in every X-ray and radiotherapy department.

It is important that student radiographers are taught how to use the equipment competently to ensure, not only the safety of the patient, but of the staff and the department. It is necessary for the student radiographers to be able to identify the component parts of the equipment and to understand their function.

The rules regarding the storage of oxygen should be known and understood. The student radiographers should be able to competently care for a patient who is receiving oxygen and should be aware of the methods of oxygen administration available. There should be an awareness of the types of patients who may require oxygen and an understanding of the observations which need to be made for these patients. It is expected that students gain practical experience in this subject whilst under experienced supervision.

Oxygen is required when the patient's normal supply of oxygen to the tissue cells cannot be maintained.

e.g. Respiratory failure
Circulatory failure
Inability of cells to combine with
oxygen (carbon monoxide poisoning)

OXYGEN SUPPLY

Piped
The pipes are clearly marked with the word oxygen

Cylinders (Fig. 15.1)
The cylinders are black with a white collar

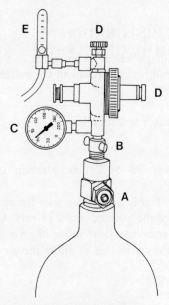

Fig. 15.1   A regulating valve on an oxygen cylinder
A – on/off switch from the cylinder
B – a locking nut for attachment to the cylinder
C – a pressure gauge – gives the pressure of oxygen in the cylinder when the
     on/off switch is open
D – valves to control the oxygen supply from the regulator to the patient
E – a flowmeter to register the rate of flow to the patient

have oxygen or 0_2 written on
are operated by a regulating valve.

MAINTENANCE AND CHECKING OF AN OXYGEN CYLINDER

The operator should check that the cylinder
   Is easily accessible
   Is easily manoeuvered
   Is periodically checked for function
   Is kept clean
   Has a disk or tear off label indicating if it is full/empty/in use
   Has a valve spanner or key available
   Has the on/off valve open

Has tubing and masks readily available
N.B. A full cylinder should always be available.

METHODS OF ADMINISTRATION

Oxygen is mixed with air before being given to a patient. If 100% oxygen is administered it could result in the patient suffering:
Pulmonary damage
Convulsions
Pain in the air sinuses and middle ear

Masks – oral/nasal

Polymasks – deliver 30–50% concentration of oxygen at 4 litres/minute (Fig. 15.2)
Disposable, light, a double bag with a wire frame, held in position by cords passed over the patients head or ears. Oxygen passes in between the layers and enters the inner bag via two holes. There are small holes in the outer bag to allow the air to mix with the oxygen.

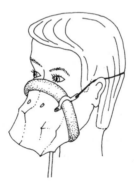

Fig. 15.2   Polymask

Edinburgh mask – delivers 35% concentration of oxygen at 3 litres/minute (Fig. 15.3)
Disposable, controlled low concentrations of oxygen administered. Air enters through the front opening. May have an attachment so that higher concentrations can be given.
Ventimasks – delivers 25% concentration of oxygen at 4 litres/minute (Fig. 15.4)
Disposable, holes round the edge to allow air to enter, have a rigid base and a flexible face area.

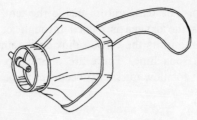

Fig. 15.3 Edinburgh mask

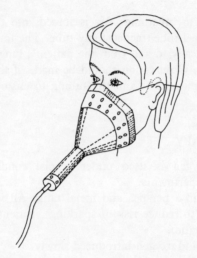

Fig. 15.4 Ventimask

Boothby, Lovelace, Bulbulian – delivers 30–40% concentration of oxygen at 4 litres/minute
Rubber mask and metal connector with a reservoir breathing bag. Patient's expired air mixes with the oxygen in the bag and the patient inspires air plus oxygen. Can be sterilised by autoclaving or gamma radiation.

Nasal tubes
Deliver 30–40% concentration of oxygen at 4 litres/minute
Two catheters are attached to a Y shaped tube, each is passed 2·5 cm along the floor of the nose. The oxygen is passed through a humidifier before being administered. Nasal tubes have the advantage that the patient can eat and drink with them in situ.

Oxygen tents
Deliver 40% concentration of oxygen at 10 litres/minute
Transparent plastic is attached to a metal frame and encloses the

patient and bed. The temperature inside the tent is 18–21°C and to maintain this the oxygen is passed through ice, or a refrigeration unit. In some units the carbon dioxide is removed by passing the air through soda lime. There are plastic zip fasteners in the sides of the tent to allow nursing procedures to be carried out.

Ventilators
For a 70 kg man, 500 ml/breath, 12 breaths/minute, therefore 6000 ml/minute.

Artificial aid to breathing. Air is forced into the lungs via a mask/endotrachael tube/tracheostomy tube. The unit pumps air or oxygen rhythmically to and from the patient's lungs. Portable units are available. Observation should be made of the patient's colour, the chest movement and the tubing to ensure that it is not trapped.

RADIOTHERAPY

Hyperbaric oxygen is used under special conditions in some radiotherapy departments.
Patient placed in a perspex and metal tank. All jewellery having been removed (to reduce risk of sparking), patient wearing a cotton gown (no static).
Tank is sealed and oxygen introduced slowly.
Pressure up to 3 atmospheres.
Oxygen tension in the blood is very high, oxygen round the tumour enhances the biological effect of radiation.
After treatment pressure is reduced slowly.
Side effects may include, fits, vomiting, earache.

Patient observations during oxygen administration
Patient's temperature, pulse and respiration rate
Colour of the patient
Signs of distress
Mask still in position
Tube supplying oxygen not kinked.

PRECAUTIONS

Oxygen itself will not burn, but it supports combustion. Therefore certain precautions must be taken to prevent fire or explosion.

No smoking
No naked lights
No electric bells or heating pads
No mechanical toys – as they may cause sparks
Care when combing patient's hair – due to static
No nylon nightwear
Patient not rubbed with oil or spirit
No oil or grease used on the cylinder fittings
If the patient has to be radiographed,
    supply turned off
    speed and care during the examination
    turn on the supply again as soon as possible.

RECORDS

Any patient receiving oxygen should have a record kept of:
    The rate of flow
    Length of time administered
    Percentage of oxygen administered.

16

Tracheostomy and suction

INTRODUCTION

A patient with a tracheostomy needs special care and attention in the Department. He needs the assurance of knowing that the staff can competently care for him and should the tracheostomy tube begin to block there will be staff present to give him assistance.

This is of particular importance to the radiotherapy staff who may be treating a patient with a tracheostomy for several weeks. If the treatment fields are in the region of the tracheostomy it is important that the students understand the necessity for replacing the silver tube for a plastic one and should know how to care for the radiation reactions around the stoma.

TRACHEOSTOMY

This is an artificial opening into the trachea in the anterior aspect of the neck to allow breathing. A tube is inserted into the opening to keep it patent (Fig. 16.1., Fig. 16.2).

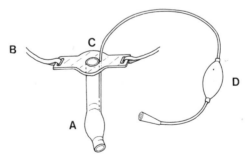

Fig. 16.1 Disposable, cuffed, tracheostomy tube
A – Inflatable cuff
B – Neck tapes
C – Opening
D – Indicating bulb, to check cuff inflated

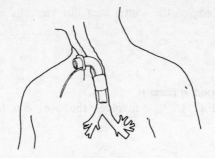

Fig. 16.2 Tracheostomy tube in position

Indications for performing a tracheostomy
Paralysis of the vocal cords/oedema of vocal cords
Obstruction of the upper respiratory tract
To allow for maximum efficiency if a ventilator is used

Patient care
Instil confidence as the patient will be apprehensive
Pencil and paper required for communication
Do not dislodge the tube
Do not remove or undo the tapes holding the tube in position
The patient should remain in the department for the minimum length of time
Do not leave the patient unattended
Have suction apparatus available

RADIOTHERAPY PATIENTS

Check that a plastic tube is used if the tracheostomy is in the treatment field
(Silver tubes produce their own characteristic radiation if irradiated)
Explain procedure carefully to the patient
Allow the patient time for communication
Give patient an alarm bell for use during treatment
Show the patient that he can be seen by the radiographers throughout the treatment
Special care should be given if the tracheostomy is recent
Keep suction apparatus close by
Check a power point is available
Stoma area should be kept free of mucus and debris

Gentle swabbing of the stoma area but vigorous washing is contraindicated.

SUCTION

Types of suction apparatus
   Portable (Fig. 16.3) – involves the use of a foot pump and catheter

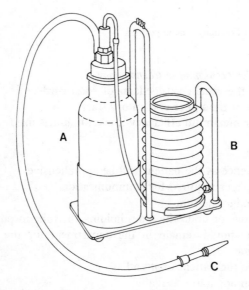

Fig. 16.3 Portable suction apparatus
A – Receiving bottle
B – Foot pump
C – Catheter attachment

   Electrical (Fig. 16.4) – mounted on casters and is plugged into the wall
   Pipeline (Fig. 16.5) – wall mounted with an independent vacuum and few controls

Use of suction
Explain the procedure to the patient
Check that the apparatus is working correctly
Clear the airway, remove patient's false teeth
Place patient supine
Cover the chest with a protective sheet
Sterile procedure

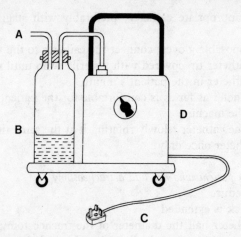

Fig. 16.4 Electrical suction apparatus
A – Catheter attachment
B – Receiving bottle
C – Electrical lead
D – Vacuum pump

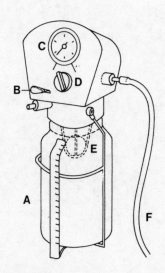

Fig. 16.5 Pipeline suction apparatus
A – Receiving bottle
B – On/off switch
C – Pressure gauge
D – Suction control
E – Float chamber
F – Tubing to catheter

Choose an appropriate catheter, preferably with staggered openings

Wearing disposable gloves, connect the catheter to the apparatus

Keep the catheter tip covered with a sterile swab until required

Place the catheter in the patient's mouth

Pass the catheter as far as is comfortable for the patient

Switch on the machine

Withdraw the catheter, slowly rotating it at the same time

Use the catheter once only.

Suction on a patient who has had a tracheostony

Sterile procedure

Patient's neck is extended

Select a catheter half the diameter of the tracheostomy tube insert into trachea, pushing gently down to the carina – procedure as above.

Throughout the procedure the colour of the patient is observed as oxygen may be required. At the end of the procedure the catheter is disposed of and the apparatus cleaned.

17

Fractures

INTRODUCTION

Radiographing bones for possible fractures may form a substantial part of a radiographer's work. They must be able to recognise the signs and symptoms associated with common fractures which could warn them of impending positioning difficulties.

A knowledge of the first aid treatment of fractures is necessary for patients admitted via the Accident and Emergency Department.

For Therapy radiographers, the most common fractures encountered will be caused by malignant deposits in the bone which may completely destroy the bone tissue in one area.

For the care of lifting and moving these patients, see Section 5 on transportation of patients.

A fracture is a break in bone continuity.

TYPES OF FRACTURE

Simple/closed Where there is no break in the skin surface
Compound/open There is a loss of continuity of the skin surface and therefore a risk of infection
Transverse (Fig. 17.1) A horizontal break

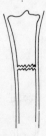

Fig. 17.1 Transverse fracture

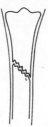

Fig. 17.2 Oblique fracture

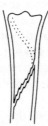

Fig. 17.3 Spiral fracture

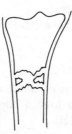

Fig. 17.4 Comminuted fracture

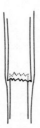

Fig. 17.5 Impacted fracture

Fig. 17.6   Compression fracture

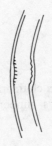

Fig. 17.7   Greenstick fracture

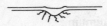

Fig. 17.8   Depressed fracture

Oblique (Fig. 17.2) An oblique break
Spiral (Fig. 17.3) Twists round, most common site is tibia
Comminuted (Fig. 17.4) Contains fragments of bone
Impacted (Fig. 17.5) The ends of the bones overlap
Compression (Fig. 17.6) The bone is crushed
Greenstick (Fig. 17.7) The bone appears bent – occurs in young children
Depressed (Fig. 17.8) Occurs when the bone (nost commonly the skull) is struck by a hard object
Pathological   Occurs because of underlying disease making the affected bone more susceptible to damage e.g. malignant tumour deposits.

Local signs and symptoms
Pain/swelling/bruising
Abnormal mobility
Deformity

Loss of use of limbs
Shortening – if occuring in a limb
Haemorrhage
Crepitus

Treatment of the fracture
Immobilise (temporary)
Reduce
Immobilise
Rehabilitate

Emergency treatment
Reassure the patient
Cover any wound with a clean cloth/arrest any haemorrhage
Immobilise with care (always supporting above and below the fracture site) by using –
  slings
  splints
  bandages
If possible, elevate a fractured limb
Treat patient for shock
Keep movement to a minimum
Nothing given by mouth

Reduction methods

Closed manipulation – a quick method usually performed under general anaesthetic, no surgery required

Mechanical traction – a slow method, performed by attaching a weight to the lower limb which slowly pulls the leg, therefore opposing the muscular pull.

Open reduction – a quick method, performed in theatre.

Immobilisation
Plaster of paris – must not be too tight. A note is made of any pain/swelling/discomfort.

Splints – can be made of aluminium with foam backing, plastic, polystyrene.

Rehabilitation
Restores normal function
Begins after reduction – the patient is encouraged to move
                    fingers/toes.

COMMON FRACTURES

Bennett's –of first metacarpal, an oblique fracture/dislocation involving the first carpo-metacarpal joint

Colles' – fracture of the lower end of radius and ulna with backward displacement of the radius

Smith's – fracture of the lower end of radius and ulna with forward displacement of the radius

March – stress fracture of a metatarsal, often a hair-line crack

Pott's – fracture/fracture dislocation of the ankle

Supracondylar – lower end of humerus, elbow is displaced backwards.

Healing of fractures

A blood clot is formed at the fracture site

The dead tissue is removed by osteoclasts

Calcium salts are deposited by osteoblasts

Callus is formed

N.B. Undue movement at an early stage is liable to delay union.

18

Haemorrhage

INTRODUCTION

It is important that student radiographers learn the treatment for haemorrhage because of the possibility of encountering a patient in the department needing immediate attention for a bleeding wound.

Diagnostic radiographers in the Accident and Emergency Department may have to radiograph patients with external bleeding but it should be stressed that a potentially more serious problem could arise if an internal haemorrhage goes unnoticed.

Radiotherapy radiographers often have to deal with patients who are suffering with haemorrhaging wounds due to tumour involvement and they are also required to assist during routine skin biopsies which frequently involve having to control a haemorrhaging wound.

Haemorrhage is the escape of blood from blood vessels, resulting from damage caused by injury or disease.

TYPES OF HAEMORRHAGE

Arterial
Blood is bright red
Spurts under pressure
Blood comes from the proximal side of the wound except where there is free anastomosis e.g. radial and ulnar arteries

Venous
Blood is dark purple
'Wells' up in an even stream
Is distal to the wound except when varicosed

Capillary
Blood is bright red

Oozes from the wound
Rarely forms large blood loss

CLASSIFICATION

Primary
Occurs at the time of injury

Reactionary
Occurs a few hours after injury and within 24 hours
Shock/drugs inhibit the blood flow

Secondary
Occurs about 10 days after injury
Is always due to sepsis

External
Blood is visible on the skin surface

Internal
No blood visible

SIGNS AND SYMPTOMS OF SEVERE HAEMORRHAGE

Rise in pulse rate
Drop in blood pressure
Pallor
Subnormal temperature
Restlessness
Rapid, sighing respiration
Skin cold, clammy
Faintness/fainting
Thirst
Dilated pupils
Pain – if bleeding into the peritoneal cavity

TREATMENT OF HAEMORRHAGE

Internal
Keep the patient warm
Lie the patient down, raise the legs, unless contraindicated
Assist if vomiting – save the vomit for inspection

Do not give the patient anything to eat or drink
Send for medical aid

External
Same general treatment as above.
In addition
  Apply digital pressure on the wound, unless a foreign body is
  present
  Cover the wound with a sterile pad
  If bleeding continues, cover the first pad with a second.
  If possible raise the limb above the level of the head (unless in-
  jury to head/neck/shoulder in which case lie the patient flat).

If a foreign body is suspected
Apply digital pressure to the nearest pressure point
for arterial bleeding – proximal to the injury
for venous bleeding – distal to the injury
N.B. A tourniquet must not be applied as this may damage
nerves, increase the blood supply and if not released may cause
gangrene.

TERMS ASSOCIATED WITH HAEMORRHAGE

Haematemesis
Vomiting of blood as a result of bleeding from the upper gastro-
intestinal tract e.g. from a gastric or duodenal ulcer. The blood
has the appearance of 'coffee grounds' when it has been in the stomach for a long time.

Haematoma
A swelling composed of blood which can occur in any part of the
body e.g. extradural – between the dura and the skull, subdural –
between the dura and the arachnoid mater, intracerebral – within
the brain.

Haematuria
Blood in the urine, can be the result of renal damage, tumour in
the renal tract or an inflammatory disorder of the urinary bladder.

Haemoptysis
Coughing up of blood from the respiratory tract as a result of car-
cinoma of the bronchus, pulmonary tuberculosis, bronchiectasis.
The blood is bright red in colour and frothy.

Haemorrhoids (piles)

Dilated veins round the anal area. Tend to be a cause of bleeding from the lower intestinal tract.

Haemothorax

Blood in the pleural cavity, associated with chest injuries e.g. fractured ribs.

19

Sterile dressings

INTRODUCTION

Diagnostic and therapeutic radiographers come into contact with open and infected wounds.

Patients involved in road traffic accidents come to Accident and Emergency departments often requiring an X-ray examination, whilst many patients are seen in the Radiotherapy department with open and infected wounds due to tumour involvement in the skin. Radiographers need to be able to set up a sterile dressings trolley or tray and apply sterile dressings in the absence of any nursing help.

This section aims at dealing with basic sterile dressing technique which should be correctly practised to prevent the spread of infection to other patients and staff and to try and keep a clean wound free from infection. Any infection in a wound will seriously delay the healing process.

DRESSINGS

Required to protect broken skin from infection

General principles
Dressing are only carried out if necessary
All instruments and dressings must be sterile
Air disturbance must be reduced to a minimum
The wound must be exposed for the minimum amount of time

DRESSING TROLLEY

Ideally, trolley settings should be done in a room reserved only for this purpose.

The trolley should be cleaned with an antiseptic solution and dried.

Top shelf (sterile items)
A sterile C.S.S.D. pack is placed on the top shelf, containing
    Gauze swabs
    Cotton wool balls
    Sterile towels or paper drapes
    Gallipots
    Sterile dressing
    4 pairs of dressing forceps

Bottom shelf (non sterile items)
Bottle of cleansing lotion eg Cetrimide 1%
Adhesive tape
Disposable bag for dirty dressings

MASKS
Usually worn to filter micro-organisms from the expired air.

Precautions
Paper masks are worn for a maximum of 10 minutes (unless they become moist, when they should be discarded)
Mask must cover the nose and mouth
The tapes only should be handled when removing the mask
Once removed the mask should be discarded – not reworn.

BASIC DRESSING PROCEDURE (NO TOUCH TECHNIQUE)
Prepare trolley
Explain the procedure to the patient
Wash hands
Open pack (handling outside only)
Pour cleansing lotion into the gallipot (not holding the bottle over the sterile area)
Remove existing dressing with forceps and dispose of dressing
Wash hands
Clean the wound — each swab only used once
                  clean from the inside to the outside by a circular/spiral movement
                  dry the area
Cover with clean dressing using sterile forceps
Attach dressing with adhesive tape or bandages
Return unused instruments and dressings to C.S.S.D. for resterilisation.

20

Diabetes

INTRODUCTION

Patients attending the X-ray or Radiotherapy departments needing regular and controlled units of insulin to keep their diabetes under control require special consideration.

It could happen that a patient accidentally forgets to administer his insulin prior to attending the hospital or misses a meal because of a delay when he arrives at the hospital. Radiographers are expected to recognise the signs and symptoms of a diabetic or insulin coma and initiate the first aid treatment if necessary.

Patients attending the department on a regular basis should, if possible, be given an appointment time which does not disrupt his own routine.

As diabetes insipidus is a completely separate disease it is necessary to be able to distinguish the differences between the two.

DIABETES MELLITUS

Beta cells of the pancreas secrete insulin which plays a part in carbohydrate metabolism. If there is a deficiency in the amount of insulin produced diabetes mellitus results.

Normal serum glucose level = 80–120mg/100ml

Diagnosis
Hyperglycaemia – excessive glucose in the blood
Glycosuria   – glucose in the urine

Signs and symptoms
Thirst
Excess urine production (contains sugar)
Weight loss

Chronic complications
Decreased arterial function (poor circulation)

Diabetic coma (hyperglycaemic coma)
Occurs if the disease is untreated or if insulin had been omitted

Signs
Slow onset
Drowsiness/unconsciousness
Deep sighing breaths
Dry skin
Smell of acetone on the breath
Fast thready pulse

Treatment
Insulin is given

Insulin coma (hypoglycaemic coma)
Caused by an overdose of insulin, or lack of food at the appropriate time

Signs and symptoms
Onset tends to be rapid
Sinking feeling and hunger
May tremble, appear drunk/confused
Shallow or normal breathing
Sweating, moist, clammy skin
No breath odour
Faintness/unconsciousness
Fast pounding pulse

Treatment
Give sugar orally or an intravenous injection of glucose is given by a medical officer

DIABETES INSIPIDUS (rare)

Occurs if the production of antidiuretic hormone which is stored in the posterior lobe of the pituitary gland, decreases.

Symptoms
Severe thirst

Passage of excessive amounts of dilute urine

THE DIABETIC PATIENT IN THE X-RAY DEPARTMENT

No special care required unless:
  Starvation required e.g. if general anaesthetic
    is required
      barium meal examinations
  Diet modification e.g. abdominal preparation

Starvation
Patient asked: to omit insulin to bring food and insulin with them
Placed first on the list
Radiologist informed

Diet modification
Only after consultation with a radiologist or the patient's general
practitioner.

THE DIABETIC PATIENT IN THE RADIOTHERAPY DEPARTMENT

Appointment given to suit the patient (not at their mealtimes)
Ambulance service should be notified if a diabetic patient is using
the transport services
Diabetic patients have an increased susceptibility to infection
which must be born in mind with radiotherapy patients
Often these patients suffer with circulatory problems and severe
arteriosclerosis, they should not be placed in cold and draughty
areas (no patient should be!)
Problems can arise if the insulin balance is upset due to patients
becoming anorexic due to the radiotherapy treatment

21

Colostomy and ileostomy

INTRODUCTION

Radiographers in the X-ray and radiotherapy department will have to deal with patients with a colostomy or ileostomy. These patients may be apprehensive of revealing their stoma to the radiographers and therefore they must receive reassurance from the radiographers that their problems will be understood and overcome.

Radiographers should know how to assist a patient with the removal of the drainage bag and be able to give advice on general management of the stoma following an X-ray examination or radiotherapy treatment, and should discuss any side effects resulting from the investigation or treatment.

COLOSTOMY/ILEOSTOMY

When a portion of either the colon (colostomy) or ileum (ileostomy) opens onto the anterior abdominal wall to form either a temporary or a permanent artificial anus (stoma) through which faeces are discharged

Indications
Rest a diseased bowel e.g. Crohn's disease
Imperforate anus
Prior to surgery or after resection of diseased bowel
e.g. Ulcerative colitis
     Diverticulosis
     Malignant tumour

Diet
Patients should avoid constipation
Fairly low residue diet required

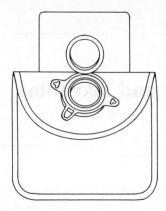

Fig. 21.1   Non drainable stoma bag

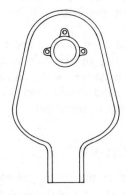

Fig. 21.2   Drainable stoma bag

Personal hygiene
Use of disposable colostomy bags (Fig. 21.1, Fig. 21.2)
Careful washing of the stoma
Use of self adhesive bags – prevent sore skin due to the indirect skin contact (see Fig 21.1)
Patient/staff wash hands before and after handling the bags

Barium enema examination
Ensure clean colostomy bag available
Enema usually performed via the stoma
Careful catheterisation of the bowel through the stoma
May require a more dilute solution
Care not to overfill bowel

Ensure facilities available for the patient with regard to hand washing and changing the bag

CARE OF THE PATIENT IN THE RADIOTHERAPY DEPARTMENT

Pelvic or abdominal irradiation may follow surgical treatment for carcinoma of the rectum if residual disease is present.

The area of the stoma is kept out of the treatment area unless there is known disease present.

Following radiotherapy diarrhoea may be a problem

Attention to diet – no foods which could enhance the problem of diarrhoea

If any anti diarrhoea drug is prescribed, care must be taken to prevent constipation

High fluid intake must be emphasised

Anti emetics required for nausea or vomiting.

22

Nursing procedures

INTRODUCTION

The general principles of nursing procedures should be taught to all hospital personnel who come into contact with patients.

Radiographing or treating hospitalised patients is only one part of the nursing programme for the patient. It is important that the care of the patient does not become isolated within individual departments of a hospital. An understanding of general nursing procedures by student radiographers will help the integration of the total nursing care for the patients.

Practical experience of these procedures should be gained on selected wards soon after the commencement of training.

BEDMAKING

Principles
To enhance patient comfort
To ensure the economical use of equipment

Articles required
Receptacles for soiled linen
Linen
    bottom sheet
    waterproof sheet
    draw sheet
    top sheet
    pillow cases
    blankets

Procedure
Clear patient's locker top
Pull out the racks on the end of the bed
Loosen the sheets
Remove blankets ·

Change the sheets
Dispose of the dirty linen
Replace the blankets
Reposition the rack
Replace articles on the locker

Patient considerations
Patient's face should never be covered by linen
Clothes should never be drawn tightly over the body

Bed accessories

Bed tables
Bed cradles – relieve pressure/weight of sheets over injured parts of the body.
Bed elevators – used to raise either end of the bed e.g. to aid breathing or as a treatment for shock.
Rings/airbeds/cushions – to reduce pressure and therefore prevent bed sores.
Ripple beds – alternate sections fill and then empty, used to prevent pressure sores.
Pulleys – enable patients on traction to lift themselves up to give themselves exercise, and makes bedmaking easier.

Continental quilts
These have now replaced 'normal' bedding in some hospitals.

Advantages
More comfortable for the patient
Create less dust therefore more hygienic
Allow easy access for nursing care
Light in weight
Easy to clean
Saves bed making time
Helps create a better atmosphere for long term residents.

Disadvantages
Some are not constructed of flame retardant material and are therefore thought to be a fire risk.

Position in bed
Supine – for relaxation, contraindications –
    Patients who are elderly
    Patients who have had abdominal surgery

Patients who are chronically ill
Prone – for spinal injuries
Semi recumbent – for medical and surgical patients
Erect, sitting – for convalescent patients
Coma position as – for unconscious patients

Dangers of bed rest
Deep vein thrombosis – changes in walls of veins causing clots, stasis of blood in the vein
Pneumonia – inflammation of lung tissue
Urinary complications – retention, infection, bedwetting
Pressure sores – areas of inflammation caused by prolonged pressure occurring usually on elbows, buttocks and heels
Semi recumbent for medical and surgical patients

PRESSURE AREA CARE

Causes of pressure sores

External

Friction	– patient being dragged over uneven surfaces
Shearing	– blood vessels are torn, can occur if the patient is scratched
Pressure	– from bony areas and contact with wet or damp surfaces and hard objects e.g. crumbs, cassettes

Internal
Old age
General health of patient
Immobility of patient
Diminished ability to appreciate pain
Pathological conditions – diabetes mellitus
                                    general paralysis

Prevention of pressure sores
Patient moved 2 hourly
Reduce pressure e.g. by using a ripple bed
Well balanced diet – high protein content
Prevent patient becoming anaemic

Treatment of pressure areas
Patient is moved 2 hourly
Use of silicon cream – protects from moisture
Use of ripple beds, water immersion beds, air rings, sheepskins

If sore develops it is treated with aseptic precautions to prevent infection

N.B. Massaging of the skin is now contraindicated as it is a form of friction and is therefore thought to encourage bed sores.

BED BATHS

Articles required
Jug of hot water
Basin
Soap
Talcum powder
Beaker, toothbrush, toothpaste, receiver
Hairbrush and comb
Nail scissors
Face and hand towels
Bath towels
Clean linen for the patient and the bed.

Patient preparation
Inform patient of procedure
Offer bedpan/urinal
Close windows
Draw bed curtains
Remove top bedclothes
Place towels over and under the patient
Remove patient's clothing

Method
Wash and dry
   face, neck, ears
   chest, arms
change the water
   lower chest, abdomen
   lower limbs
   back
   genital region – washed by patient if possible
Talcum powder is applied

Additional care
Nails cut if required
Hair washed if necessary
Teeth cleaned

After care
Patient dresses in clean clothes
Bed is remade
Drink is given
Windows are opened
Curtains drawn back

MOUTH CARE

Complications of mouth neglect
Crustations on lips and teeth
Cracked lips
Furring of the tongue
Herpes – mouth sores
Odious taste
Can destroy sense of taste
Halitosis – bad breath

Can lead to infection of
Stomach   – gastritis
Lungs   – inhalation pneumonia
Middle ear   – otitis media
Parotid gland   – parotitis
Tonsils   – tonsillitis
Tongue   – glossitis

Cleansing by the patient
Clean the teeth
Clean dentures with warm water and cleansing
powder
Mouth wash given

To cleanse a patient's mouth
Remove dentures
Clean the dentures with a brush
Swab mouth with liquid
Clean teeth from gum to crown
Give a mouth wash

BEDPANS AND URINALS

Giving a bedpan
Place screens round the patient

Ensure the bedpan is warm and dry
Take the pan to the patient covered
Lift the patient if necessary
Adjust and support the patient if necessary
Cleanse the patient using toilet tissue or swabs

Emptying the bedpan
Inspect the contents for blood, unusual colour
Flush the pan
Inspect to see if clean
Sterilise if necessary

Disposable bedpans
Strengthened cardboard (papiére mâche)
Support for the bedpan is required – in the form of a metal frame
After use inspect contents
Dispose of pan and contents

Urinals
Take the urinal to the patient covered
Assist if necessary
Check contents for blood etc.
Record the volume of urine if necessary
Disinfect or sterilise the urinal
Place the urinal upside down to drain

LUMBAR PUNCTURE

Indications
To remove cerebro-spinal fluid for analysis
To measure the pressure of cerebro-spinal fluid
To introduce a contrast agent to examine the nerve roots and spinal canal

Equipment –sterile procedure
Swabs/skin cleanser
Syringe
Needles
Local anaesthetic
Lumbar puncture needle
Manometer
Sterile specimen bottle

Contrast agent
Sterile towels

Procedure
Patient lies on his side
Hips and knees flexed
Skin cleaned
Local anaesthetic introduced over the site of the puncture
Lumbar puncture needle introduced between 2nd and 3rd lumbar
vertebra, (below termination of the spinal cord)

Investigations

> *Pressure*   – taken with a manometer attached to the needle
> (normal 75–150 mm)
> *Sample*   – a small quantity of cerebro-spinal fluid is collected
> in the specimen bottle and is sent for analysis
> *Radiography* – contrast agent is introduced during myelography
> or radiculography

23

Temperature, pulse, respiration and blood pressure

INTRODUCTION

When dealing with physically sick patients it is often necessary to carry out an accurate assessment of a patient's physical condition. An indication of how ill a patient is can be found by taking a patient's temperature, pulse and respiration. The radiographer is often the person having the immediate contact with the patient which means she is the person who has to make the preliminary assessment of that patient.

Student radiographers should gain practical experience in these skills on the ward and in the department.

TEMPERATURE

Features of a typical clinical thermometer (Fig. 23.1)
10 cm long graduated glass tube with a 'bulb' at one end
A magnifying lens on one side

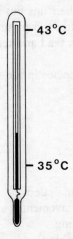

Fig. 23.1 Clinical thermometer

A short temperature range, usually 35°C–43°C
Mercury filled bulb and central column
Can be sterilised using chemical solutions
Unfortunately is breakable
Constriction above the bulb to retain the position of the mercury
Self registering
Accurate if used correctly

N.B. A rectal thermometer has a wider, alcohol filled, bulb which is either blue, or has a blue dot to identify it.

General principles

Temperature should not be taken directly after
  a hot bath
  a hot drink
  smoking
Temperature may be taken
  orally
  rectally
  in axilla/groin
Patient has his own thermometer which is wiped with swabs before use. An explanation is given to the patient regarding the procedure.

Orally

Thermometer is shaken to read below 35·5°C
Thermometer is placed under the patient's tongue
Patient is asked to close their lips but not bite
Thermometer is left in situ for 5 minutes
Remove the thermometer, read and record immediately
Shake mercury down
Wipe thermometer and replace in the disinfectant.

Contraindications

  Infants
  Unconscious patients
  Delirious patients
  Insane patients
  Patients who suffer from epilepsy
  If mouth closure is inconvenient – e.g. cough
  obstructed nasal breathing
  dyspnoea (difficult breathing)

Rectally
(The normal reading is 2° higher than skin temperature and 1° higher than oral temperature)
The thermometer has a wider bulb which is coloured and filled with alcohol

Method
Thermometer is shaken to read below 35°C
The bulb is lubricated
Patient lies on their side
Thermometer is inserted 5 cm into the rectum
Thermometer is left in situ for 5 minutes
Read and record immediately
Clean the thermometer

Axilla/groin
The normal reading is 1° less than oral and 2° less than rectal temperature.

Method
The skin surfaces must be dry
The thermometer is shaken to read below 35°C
The thermometer is placed under the axilla or in the groin
Skin surfaces are pressed together to exclude air
Thermometer is left in situ for 5 minutes
Read and record immediately
Clean the thermometer

Digital thermometers
Used for oral, arm and skin temperatures
Rectal probes are available
Overall range 20–50°C
10-20 second response time
Temperature on a digital display
Display can be 'held' for reference purposes
Battery operated

Electronic thermometers(Fig 23.2)
Similar to digital but with a meter display
Disposable probe covers are available
5 second response time
If probe covers used, 9–12 second response time

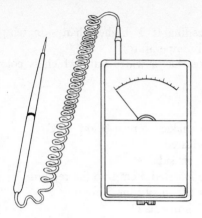

Fig. 23.2 Electronic thermometer

Probe sterilised with alcohol
Battery operated.

Recording the temperature

The temperature is recorded on the patient's chart (Fig 23.3) with a dot which is joined to the previous dot with either a straight line if it is above or below the previous reading, or a loop if the previous reading is the same. The thermometer should always be read in good light and recording must be done immediately.

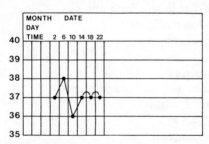

Fig. 23.3 Temperature chart

PULSE

Each pulse represents a cardiac cycle and can be felt where an artery passes superficially and lies over a bone i.e. at a pressure point.

Common sites
Radial pulse –wrist

Femoral pulse – groin
Carotid pulse – neck

Checking the pulse rate (radial)
Explain the procedure to the patient
Ensure the patient is at rest
The hand and arm should be supported
Place your fingers (not the thumb as there is a pulse in the thumb) over the pulse to be recorded
If regular count the beats for 30 seconds
Double the number and record immediately
If irregular the beats are counted for a full minute

Electronic pulse monitor (Fig 23.4)
A spring-loaded photocell is clipped on the finger
A diode lamp flashes with the pulse rate
Scale measurement range 30-200 beats/minute
10 second response time
Battery operated

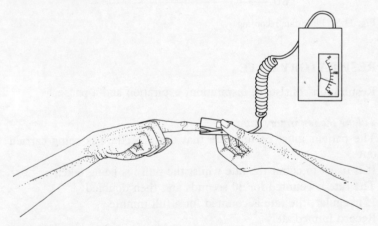

Fig. 23.4 Electronic pulse monitor

In addition to the rate, note the
Tension – bounding/thready
Rhythm – regular/irregular
Volume – full/normal/small

In a normal pulse the
Rate   – corresponds to the age of the patient

Rhythm – regular
Volume – moderate
Tension – not easily compressed

Recording the pulse rate

The pulse is recorded immediately on the patient's chart
(Fig. 23.5) with a dot which is joined to the previous dot with
either a straight line if it is above or below the previous reading, or
a loop if the previous reading is the same.

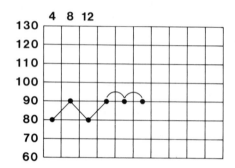

Fig. 23.5   Pulse rate recording

RESPIRATORY RATE

Respiration consists of inspiration, expiration and a pause.

Taking the respiratory rate
The patient must be unaware that the procedure is being carried
out
It is usual to count the rate whilst the pulse is being taken
The rate is counted for 30 seconds and then doubled
If irregular, the rate is counted for a full minute
Record immediately

In addition to the rate, note the
    Depth of respiration
    Regularity
    Rhythm

Recording the respiratory rate

The respiratory rate is recorded immediately on the patient's chart
(Fig 23.6) with a dot which is joined to the previous dot with

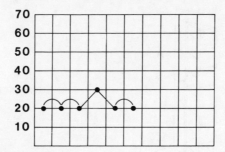

Fig. 23.6 Respiratory rate recording

either a straight line if it is above or below the previous reading, or a loop if the previous reading is the same.

BLOOD PRESSURE

Factors maintaining blood pressure:
 Pumping force of the heart
 Quantity of blood in the body
 Elasticity of the blood vessels
 Resistance to the passage of blood in the vessels
 Viscosity of the blood

Manual sphygmomanometer (Fig 23.7)

Instrument used to measure blood pressure which consist of a:
 Mercury manometer in millimetres
 Collapsible arm band
 Pump and valve
Also required is a stethoscope.

Method of taking blood pressure
Patient should be at rest
Patient extends their arm and it is supported
Arm band is placed round the patient's arm, above the elbow
Arm band is inflated
The radial pulse is palpated during inflation
Remember the level of mercury when the pulse disappears
The arm band is inflated for a further 5 millimetres
Place the stethoscope below the crease of the elbow
Release the air from the arm band until the first sound is heard
The level of mercury gives the systolic pressure (when the chambers of the heart are full blood)

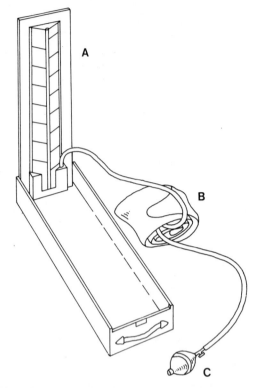

Fig. 23.7 Manual sphygmomanometer
A — Graduated mercury column
B — Inflatable arm band
C — Hand pump

Listen until the sound reaches the maximum
1 soft sound followed by a second soft sound is then heard
The level of mercury gives the diastolic pressure (when the heart relaxes)

Electronic sphygmomanometer (Fig 23.8)
No stethoscope required
Cuff placed round the arm, 4-5 cm above the antecubital fossa
Cuff inflated by repeatedly squeezing the bulb
Cuff automatically deflates and manometer needle drops
First flash/bleep denotes systolic pressure
Unit continues to flash and bleep with the blood pressure sounds
Last flash/bleep indicates the diastolic pressure

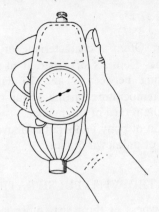

Fig. 23.8   Electronic sphygmomanometer

Battery powered
Dial range 20-200 mm of mercury

Recording the blood pressure

The blood pressure is recorded immediately on the patient's chart
(Fig 23.9), usually at right angles to the other readings. A straight
line joins the diastolic and the systolic pressures.

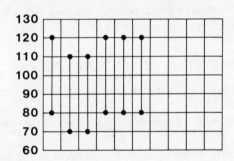

Fig. 23.9   Blood pressure recording

TERMS ASSOCIATED WITH TEMPERATURE

Fever. Pyrexia 37·2°C–40·5°C.

Hyperpyrexia. A dangerous condition with high body temperature above 40·5°C.

Hypothermia. General lowering of body temperature, may occur
when heat loss exceeds heat production. Result following shock or
injury, fatal if uncontrolled. Temperatures are usually below 35°C
and therefore a special thermometer 24°C–41°C is required.

Normal. 35·5°C–37·2°.

Subnormal. Below 35°C.

Pel-Ebstein fever: Often a characteristic of Hodgkin and non Hodgkin lymphoma. Consists of a period of pyrexia – often as high as 40°C lasting between 3 and 10 days, followed by a period of normal temperature lasting about the same length of time, followed by the return of the pyrexia.

Pyrexia: Elevation of body temperature above normal.

P.U.O: Pyrexia of unknown origin.

TERMS ASSOCIATED WITH PULSE RATE

Bradycardia: Slowness of the heart, pulse less than 60/minute, can occur during sleep/old age/hypothermia, or as a result of treatment by certain drugs.

Normal: Adults – 65 to 80 beats/minute (women 5 beats faster than men)

New born infant – 120 to 140 beats/minute

Child age 5 – 100 beats/minute

Old age – Pulse slows

Very old age – Pulse quickens

Tachycardia: Increase in heart beat above normal limits, pulse rate 160 – 200 beats/minute occurs following shock/haemorrhage/heart condition/hyperthermia/action of certain drugs.

TERMS ASSOCIATED WITH RESPIRATION

Apnoea. Associated with dyspnoea, absence of breathing for short periods.

Asthma. Gasping for breath due to spasm of the muscle walls of the bronchi.

Bronchiectasis. Abnormally dilated bronchi in the lungs, patient therefore prone to bronchial obstruction.

Cheyne-Stokes respiration. A cyclic pattern of irregular breathing occuring in patients with cerebral disease especially where there is raised intracranial pressure. Slow and shallow to start, progressing in speed and depth to a maximum then depressed again, finally there is a period of apnoea for about 15 seconds and the cycle begins again.

Dyspnoea. Difficulty in breathing e.g. obstruction of airway, can be caused by heart disease. Patients are nursed semirecumbant.

Haemoptysis. Coughing up of blood from the respiratory tract.
Normal respiration rate 20 breaths/minute.
Sighing. Long slow inspiration followed by rapid expiration.
Stertorous. Breathing noisy, cheeks puffed in and out with each breath.
Wheezing. Rattling noises occur when air is forced through fluid.

TERMS ASSOCIATED WITH BLOOD PRESSURE

C.C.F: Congestive cardiac failure.
Hypertension: High blood pressure (can be due to renal disease) caused by narrowing of arteries causing resistance to peripheral circulation.
Hypotension: Low blood pressure.
Normal blood pressure. $\frac{120}{80}$ $\left(\frac{\text{Systolic}}{\text{Diastolic}}\right)$

Infancy: 50 (Diastolic) 70 – 90 (Systolic)
Childhood: 60 (Diastolic) 80 – 100 (Systolic)
Adolescence: 60 (Diastolic) 90 – 110 (Systolic)
Young adult: 60 – 70 (Diastolic) 110 – 125 (Systolic)
Adult: 80 – 90 (Diastolic) 130 – 150 (Systolic)

24

Catheterisation and intubation

INTRODUCTION

Although it is unlikely that a student radiographer will have to catheterise a patient there will be occasions when they will have to radiograph or treat patients with urinary catheters in situ.

During certain diagnostic examinations the student may have to assist in the catheterisation of patients and it is therefore important that they understand the principles of catheterisation.

A chart outlining some of the more common catheters is available for reference purposes.

CATHETERISATION

The introduction of a tube into the body for the purpose of:
  Discharging the fluid contents of a cavity
  Establishing the patency of a canal
  Introducing an agent into a cavity

INTUBATION

The introduction of a tube into a hollow organ to keep it open e.g. into the larynx to ensure the passage of air, in general anaesthesia.

Introduction of a catheter
Catheterisation of the bladder is a sterile procedure and care must be taken:
  Not to introduce micro organisms
  Not to damage the urethra

Female patients
Urethral opening is swabbed
Using sterile gloves, or forceps, the catheter is introduced about 5 cm into the urethra

The catheter is attached to the patient's thigh, to prevent it from becoming dislodged

Male patients
The urethral opening is cleaned
The urethra is anaesthetised (lignocaine gel)

   After 5 minutes
The catheter is introduced using an aseptic technique
The catheter is attached to the patient's thigh

If the catheter becomes displaced
Do not reinsert as this will contaminate the bladder
Report the occurrence

If the catheter comes out
Do not reinsert
Report the occurrence

Disposable catheters

Advantages
Hygenic
Time saving
Readily available
Conveniently disposed of

Disadvantages
Large supplies are required
Disposal must be efficient
Cannot be tested prior to use

Foley catheters (Fig. 24.1)
Can be used on radiotherapy wards for patients with dysuria

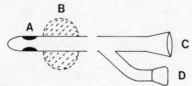

Fig. 24.1   Foley catheter
   A – Eyelet
   B – Inflatable balloon
   C – For urinary bag attachment
   D – Side tube for inflating the balloon

Patients with carcinoma of the bladder are catheterised prior to performing a localising cystogram.

If difficulties are expected during the treatment e.g. dysuria, then the catheter may be left in place until the patient is able to pass urine easily.

Principle of catheter insertion is the same as before, but the balloon, found at the proximal end of the catheter, is inflated with sterile water or air which keeps the catheter in place.

TYPES OF CATHETERS/TUBES

Name	Material	Use	Sterilisation method
Drainage tubes	Rubber	Draining body cavities	Autoclaving
Foley catheter	Silicone	Bladder intubation (self retaining)	Autoclaving
Franklin catheter	Soft rubber	Rectal intubation	Autoclaving
Jaques'	Soft rubber	Rectal intubation	Autoclaving
Jaques' (disposable)	Polythene	Bladder intubation	Gamma radiation
Kifa (disposable)	Polythene	Aortography	Gamma radiation
Magill's laryngeal & bronchial tubes	Polythene	Bronchography Resuscitation	Gamma radiation
Nasal catheter	Rubber	Bronchography Oxygen administration	Autoclaving
Oesophageal tube (disposable)	Polythene	Gastric feeds Duodenal/small bowel intubation	Gamma radiation
Rectal cathether	Soft rubber	Rectal intubation	Autoclaving
Ryle's tube (disposable)	Polythene	Duodenal/small bowel intubation	Gamma radiation
Tiemann's catheter	Soft rubber	Male bladder catheterisation	Autoclaving
Ureteric catheter	Polythene	Retrograde pyelogram	Gamma radiation

25

Fire procedure

INTRODUCTION

Whatever the nature of employment in the Health Service it is directed to the support and protection of the existence and well being of human life. A knowledge of how to prevent fire and what action to take in the event of fire is very necessary for all hospital staff. Staff are required to attend lectures and fire drills under the provision of the Fire Precautions Act 1971.

This section on fire safety is therefore intended to be complementary to training which is received in the hospital. The traditional approach to fire protection is to identify and seek to eliminate the causes of fire, or failing that, to detect a fire as early as possible and contain it whilst it is being extinguished.

MAJOR CAUSES OF FIRE IN A DEPARTMENT

Misuse of electricity
Sunshine and matches
Faults in heating systems
Spontaneous combustion
Improper refuse disposal

The major hazard for radiographers is the electrical fire. With few exceptions, fires of electrical origin occur due to lack of reasonable care in the use or maintenance of electrical installations and apparatus. The power used in radiographic equipment is capable of igniting insulation or other combustibles if the equipment is not adequate to carry the load or is not properly used, installed and maintained.

Common causes of electrical fires
Failure of insulation giving rise to short circuits or earth faults
Overheating of cables or equipment
Ignition of flammable substances by electrostatic discharge

The second major hazard is film storage, although X-ray film is classed as non-flammable it has a combustibility similar to that of paper with the additional danger of dense volumes of carbon monoxide and other toxic gases.

FIRE PREVENTION

Be familiar with the local fire procedure
Ensure fire doors are not obstructed
Know the position of fire alarms
Know the position of the nearest fire appliances

Types of appliance available

Black extinguisher – carbon dioxide – electrical fires
Red extinguisher   – water   – 'normal' fires
Blue extinguisher – dry powder   – all types of fire
Hose   – water   – 'normal' fires

FIRE ROUTINE

Break glass on fire alarm
Remove patient from the room
Switch off the mains supply if possible
For X-ray equipment, use a black fire extinguisher, aimed at base of fire
If smoke present – keep low
When leaving the room ensure that the doors and windows are closed

Operation of equipment

Black, carbon dioxide cylinder
   Hold neck (not the handle)
   Remove the pin
   Direct the nozzle at the fire
   Firmly squeeze the handle

Red, water cylinder
   Place cylinder on the floor 4 metres from the fire
   Kneel beside the cylinder
   Hold the nozzle firmly
   Remove the safety device
   Strike (do not press) the knob
   Aim at the base of the fire

Hose
   Turn on at the wall
   Take to the fire (4 metres distant)
   Turn on
   Aim at the base of the fire

Remember
Fire is an alarming threat in any situation. In a hospital where the safety and lives of colleagues and often helpless patients are at stake, it can be terrifying and tragic. The dangers and ill effects of smoke cannot be over-emphasized. Prevention is the first and best precaution, be constantly alert for fire risks of any kind.

Glossary

Abscess   a cavity which contains pus
Allergy   reaction to a substance eg iodine
Ambulent   walking
Amnesia   loss of memory
Ampoule   container, usually glass, for sterile solutions
Anaesthetic   drug producing loss of feeling
Analgesic   drug which relieves pain
Aneurysm   abnormal dilation of an artery
Anorexia   loss of appetite
Antibiotic   substance used to fight against infection
Antibody   substance either natural or introduced that helps protect the body from infection
Antiemetic   agent which prevents nausea and vomiting
Antihistamine   substance introduced to counteract an allergy
Antiseptic   agent that stops or inhibits the growth of bacteria but does not necessarily kill them
Anuria   arrest of urinary output
Aperient   mild drug given to produce peristaltic action and therefore bowel emptying
Apnoea   cessation of breathing
Arterial haemorrhage   bleeding from an artery
Arthritis   inflammation of a joint
Arthrodesis   fusion of a joint, usually by surgical means
Ascites   accumulation of serous fluid in the peritoneal cavity
Asepsis   exclusion of micro-organisms
Asphyxia   unconsciousness resulting from lack of oxygen
Atresia   closure of normal opening or canal e.g. oesophageal atresia in infants
Autoclave   equipment for sterilising articles e.g. by using steam under pressure
Bacteria   infective micro-organism
Barrier nursing   method of nursing an infectious patient
Bedpan   a portable receptacle for receiving urine and faeces

Bed Sore   an ulcer usually caused by lack of blood supply to an area

Biopsy   removal of tissue from the living to determine the histology

Biopsy forceps   instruments which can be used to perform a biopsy

Blood count   measure of the number of erythrocytes, thrombocytes, platelets and leucocytes per cubic millimetre of blood (per litre of blood)

Blood pressure   pressure of blood against walls of blood vessels/heart

Blood sugar   amount of carbohydrate in the blood, measure of glucose level

Bradycardia   slow heartbeat

Bronchoscopy   examination, by visual inspection of the bronchus using a bronchoscope

Brook Airway   instrument used for expired air resuscitation

Burn   injury by dry heat

Cachexia   wasting away of the body usually associated with malignant disease

Calculi   small mineral deposits usually found in the biliary or renal tract

Cannula   hollow tube inserted into a body cavity for the introduction of substances

Cardiac arrest   cessation of cardiac output

Catheter   tube for introduction of fluid into the body or the discharge of substances e.g. urine

Catheterization   insertion of a catheter

Cathetron unit   remote controlled unit for placing radioactive Cobalt into the cervix and uterus

Cautery   instrument to coagulate blood vessels or destroy tissue by chemical means or heat

Claustrophobia   fear of confined spaces

Colic   acute abdominal pain usually associated with biliary or renal calculi blocking a duct

Colonic washout   method of clearing the bowel of faecal matter

Colostomy   artificial anus on anterior abdominal wall

Coma   unconsciousness from which the patient cannot be aroused

Comatose   being in a coma

Comminuted fracture   a break in the bone where the bone is fragmented

Complicated fracture   a break in the bone with associated blood vessel or nerve injury

Compound dislocation   joint dislocation where there is an external wound communicating with the joint

Compound fracture   when part of the fracture is in contact with the external surface of the body

Compression band   immobilisation device which also displaces body tissue laterally and therefore enables a reduction in radiographic exposure to be made

Compression bandage   a bandage applied over cotton wool pads, to joints to help to reduce infusion into the joint space

Concussion   a state resulting from the brain being shaken violently

Contrast agent   a drug introduced into the body for diagnostic purpose to outline a space or organ

Contusion   injury by a blow when the skin is not broken e.g. a bruise

Cross infection   infection that a patient receives from another person

Cryosurgery   destruction of diseased tissue by freezing, without harming adjacent tissue

Cyanosis   a bluish tinge to the skin due to lack of oxygen

Cytotoxic drugs   drugs which inhibit the growth of cells

Diabetic   a person suffering from diabetes

Diabetic coma   unconsciousness due to lack of insulin

Diathermy   use of heat to coagulate tissues

Disinfectant   agent that destroys or inhibits the growth of micro-organisms

Dislocation   displacement of one or more bones with relation to each other

Disposable items   articles which are only used once and then discarded, reduces crossinfection

Diuresis   increased excretion of urine

Drug   a substance used as a medicine

Dyspepsia   disturbed digestion

Dysphagia   difficulty in swallowing

Dysphonia   difficulty in speaking

Dyspnoea   difficulty in breathing

Dystrophy   degeneration

Dysuria   painful or difficult urination

Emetic   a drug used to induce vomiting

Enema   a rectal injection of fluid

Epilation   loss of hair

Epilepsy   brain disorder which produces fits

Epileptic   a person who suffers from epilepsy

Epistaxis nosebleed

Erythema redness of the skin

Filamented swab swab used in surgery with a radiopaque thread so it can be detected radiographically if necessary

Fistula an abnormal passage between two organs

Flatulence excessive gas in the stomach and intestinal tract

Fracture a break in bone continuity

General anaesthesia total loss of consciousness and therefore insensitive to pain

Gram stain – positive, organisms retain staining solution negative, organisms lose staining solution and will take up counter stain

Greenstick fracture incomplete break of the bone in young children

Haematemesis vomiting of blood

Haematoma a swelling due to a collection of blood

Haematuria blood in the urine

Haemoptysis coughing up of blood

Haemorrhoids collection of blood vessels at the anus – piles

Hemiplegia paralysis of one side of the body

Histology study of cells, organs and tissues

Hormone chemical which acts on organs remote from its origin

Hyperglycaemic coma (Diabetic coma) excess of sugar in the blood causing loss of consciousness

Hyperpyrexia high temperature over 40.6°C

Hypertension high blood pressure

Hypochondriac person who thinks they are ill when they are not

Hypodermic beneath the skin

Hypoglycaemic low level of sugar in the blood

Hypotension low blood pressure

Hypothermia low body temperature below 35°C

Immunisation introduction of antibodies to protect a person from disease

Impaction when one aspect of a bone is growing into another. When one fragment of fractured bone is driven into another

Incontinence inability to control the evacuation of faeces/urine

Infection invasion of a person or object by organisms e.g. bacteria

Inflammation reaction of tissues to injury

Infusion introduction of a liquid into the body over a long period of time

Injection introducing a liquid into the body via a needle

Insomnia sleeplessness

Insulin coma unconsciousness as a result of an overdose of insulin

Intravenous injection injection into a vein

Ischaemia diminished blood supply

Laryngeal mirror mirror for inspecting oral cavity and larynx

Laxative agent to relieve constipation

Leukaemia cancer of the blood forming white cells

Leucocytosis increase in the total number of white blood cells

Leucopenia decrease in the number of leucocytes in the blood

Local anaesthetic a drug used to render a specific area of the body insensitive to pain

Malignant growth a growth which if not checked will spread locally, usually metastasize and eventually terminate in death

Mastectomy surgical removal of a breast

Medicine a substance used for treating disease

Menorrhagia excessive menstrual flow

Metastasis a secondary tumour produced by a malignant primary tumour

Necrosis death of tissue

Neoplasm new growth

Nephritis inflammation of the kidney

Neuralgia pain in a nerve

Neurosis abnormal anxiety

Obese overweight (excessive)

Oedema collection of lymph causing swelling

Opaque media contrast agents

Opaque medium contrast agent

Ophthalmoscope instrument for examining the interior of the eye

Osteoporosis deossification of bone

Osteosclerosis increased density of bone

Palliative relieves symptoms but does not cure

Paralysis loss of muscle function and sensation

Paraparesis partial paralysis of lower limbs

Paraplegic person with paralysis of the lower limbs

Parenternal outside the alimentary tract, injection through the skin

Pathogen agent capable of producing disease

Pathological condition condition caused by disease

Polyuria passage of excessive quantities of urine

Post anaesthesia after anaesthetic and before full recovery

Premedication drug given prior to an anaesthetic to calm the patient

Pressure point place where a pulse is felt – where a superficial artery crosses a bone

Pressure sore an ulcer caused by lack of blood supply to an area

Proctitis inflammation of the anus or rectum

Prolapse the sinking down of an organ eg rectum, uterus

Prophylactic agent which prevents the development of a disease

Pulmonary embolism blockage of a blood vessel in the lungs

Pulse rate number of cardiac contractions per minute

Purgative a strong drug to encourage complete bowel evacuation

Pyrexia fever

Respiratory rate number of breaths per minute

Resuscitation restoration of life after apparent death

Retention of urine inability to pass urine

Reverse Barrier Nursing special nursing procedure when a person is prone to infection

Rubor redness due to inflammation

Scald injury caused by moist heat

Scalpel a surgical knife

Sedation state induced by a drug to calm and allay pain

Shock a condition when there is insufficient blood to fill the major arteries

Sinus an abnormal passage opening on the skin surface

Sphygmomanometer instrument for measuring blood pressure

Sterile free from micro-organisms

Sterilisation to render free from micro-organisms

Stupor when a person is partly conscious but can be roused

Subluxation partial dislocation

Suction apparatus for removing secretions

Surgical mask a mask to cover the nose and mouth to prevent the contamination of a sterile area by droplet infection

Symptoms an indication of a particular disorder of which the patient complains

Syndrome a group of symptoms which characterise a disease or lesion

Syringe instrument for holding fluid for injection

Tachycardia rapid heart beat

Tracheostomy artificial opening in the trachea or insertion of a tube, to maintain breathing

Unconscious a lack of awareness, with no reflexes

Urinal a vessel for receiving urine

Urinary catheter   catheter inserted into the urinary bladder to drain urine

Venous haemorrhage   bleeding from a vein

Vomit bowl   receptacle to receive vomit

Index